Certified Coding Specialist (CCS) Review Guide

2009

Jennifer Hornung Garvin,
PhD, RHIA, CPHQ, CCS, CTR, FAHIMA

AHIMA
American Health Information Management Association®

ISBN 978-1-58426-236-7

AHIMA Product No. AC400409

AHIMA Staff:
Melanie Endicott, MBA/HCM, RHIA, CCS, CCS-P, Technical Reviewer
Karen Kostick, RHIT, CCS, CCS-P, Technical Reviewer
Katherine Greenock, Editorial and Production Coordinator
Ashley Sullivan, Assistant Editor
Pamela Woolf, Developmental Editor
Ken Zielske, Director of Publications

American Health Information Management Association
233 North Michigan Avenue, 21st Floor
Chicago, Illinois 60601-5800
http://www.ahima.org

Contents

About the Author

Jennifer Hornung Garvin, PhD, RHIA, CPHQ, CCS, CTR, FAHIMA is currently a Health Research Science Specialist at the Salt Lake City VA IDEAS Research Center and an Assistant Professor at the University of Utah School of Medicine in the Division of Clinical Epidemiology. She is a Health Information Management (HIM) professional with more than 24 years of experience in HIM and medical informatics. She received an associate of science and a post-baccalaureate certificate in HIM from Gwynedd-Mercy College, bachelor and doctoral degrees from Temple University, a master's degree in business (MBA) from St. Josephs University, and a graduate certificate in Biomedical Informatics from the Oregon Health and Science University. Her professional training includes a postdoctoral fellow at the Center for Health Equity Research and Promotion (CHERP) sponsored by the Department of Veteran Affairs (VA) at the Philadelphia VA Medical Center (PVAMC) in association with the University of Pennsylvania School of Medicine (SOM).

She was the program director of AHIMA accredited associate and bachelor degrees as well as an AHIMA approved coding certificate program at Gwynedd-Mercy College for nine years before seeking research training. Dr. Garvin served on the AHIMA Board of Directors, as Chair of the Research Committee, and as President of Pennsylvania Health Information Management Association (PHIMA) and the Lehigh Valley Health Information Management Association (LVHIMA) among other HIM volunteer leadership roles. She is currently serving on the AHIMA Quality Initiatives and Secondary Data Practice Council. She champions the need for quality data to improve health.

Acknowledgments

The author wishes to thank the following individuals for being editors, reviewers, and publishers of past editions of the *CCS Exam Success Review Book:*

Elizabeth Layman, PhD, RHIA, CCS, FAHIMA
Kathy Arner, LPN, RHIT, CCS, CPC
Genevive Badroe
Christine Staropoli, MS, RHIA, CCS
Angela Picard Carney, PhD, RHIA
Stephen Weiner, DO
Julian Wade Farrior, PhD
Pam Farrior, RPh
Aileen Stanton, CHCO, CCS, CCP
Pauline Benson, RHIT, CHCO, CCS, CCP
Becky Thorson, RHIT, CCS
Linda Donahue, RHIT, CCS, CCS-P, CPC
Christina Benjamin, RHIA, CSS, CSS-P

And any other reviewers from past editions who were inadvertently not named.

In addition a special thank you goes to all the HIM professionals who have sent me questions and suggestions regarding the contents of this book. You have made this work extra special.

I also so much appreciate the helpful AHIMA publication staff members who have assisted the production of this text.

About the CD-ROM

The CD-ROM accompanying this book contains skill building multiple choice questions and a 60-question multiple choice practice exam that can be run in practice or exam simulation mode. The CD-ROM will run on Windows versions 98 or later.

To install the practice exams on your computer:

1. Insert the CD-ROM in your computer's CD/DVD drive.
2. Double-click the .exe file.
3. When asked if you would like to extract files from this archive, select Yes.
4. Accept the license agreement.
5. If offered an installation path, choose the default path suggested.
6. A message will appear stating that the files have been successfully extracted.
7. The Setup Wizard will open.
8. Follow on-screen instructions through setup and installation.

The exam simulation is written for a Microsoft Windows environment. To run the test simulations on a Macintosh, you will need to simulate a Windows environment using additional software for a Mac, such as Apple's Bootcamp. AHIMA cannot guarantee this CD will run on a Mac.

Windows Vista users: right-click the program icon and then click **Run as administrator**.

This software product is designed to work on Windows 2000, XP and Vista. Under most circumstances, installation will be easy. Double click the program icon to begin the installation.

Windows Vista users may get an error message on installation. **Windows Vista users must right click on the _.exe file icon and select "run as administrator".** The program should then extract and install.

However, in some controlled environments (such as corporate environments, where users are locked down), the process gets a bit more complex.

As part of the install process, some dll and ocx files are silently registered into the system registry. This process requires admin rights, so in some cases, end users may need to have their privileges elevated to install, but afterwards, they will not need to have admin rights to actually use the software.

In **Windows Vista**, users without admin rights will automatically be prompted for the admin password during the installation, *but*, if the user does not have admin rights, the application, and the shortcuts to the application will not be created on their account (but instead, on the admin users account). This is obviously not the desired result, but is a consequence of the way Vista works.

About the CCS Exam

Coding professionals who pass the Certified Coding Specialist (CCS) exam are professionals skilled in classifying medical data from patient records, generally in the hospital setting. These coding practitioners review patients' records and assign numeric codes for each diagnosis and procedure. To perform this task, they must possess expertise in the ICD-9-CM and CPT coding systems. In addition, the CCS is knowledgeable of medical terminology, disease processes, and pharmacology. Hospitals or medical providers report coded data to insurance companies, or to the government in the case of Medicare and Medicaid recipients, for reimbursement of expenses. Researchers and public health officials also use coded medical data to monitor patterns and explore new interventions. Coding accuracy is thus highly important to healthcare organizations because of its impact on revenues and describing health outcomes, and in fact, certification is becoming an implicit industry standard. Accordingly, the CCS credential demonstrates tested data quality and integrity skills in a coding practitioner. The CCS certification examination assesses mastery proficiency in coding rather than entry-level skills. Professionals experienced in coding inpatient and outpatient records should consider obtaining this certification.

To be eligible to sit for the CCS examination, candidates must have earned a high school diploma from a United States high school or have an equivalent educational background. Although not required, it is strongly recommended that candidates have at least three years of on-the-job experience in:

- Hospital-based inpatient coding for multiple case types (for example, circulatory, pregnancy, neoplasms, genitourinary, musculoskeletal, respiratory, and endocrine, nutritional and metabolic diseases, and immunity disorders)
- Hospital-based ambulatory/outpatient care coding for multiple case types (for example, eye, musculoskeletal, integumentary, ENT, injury and poisoning, cardiac cath, interventional radiology, and pain management)

  and

- Completed coursework in anatomy and physiology, pathophysiology, and pharmacology, or demonstrated proficiency in these areas

The multiple choice items on the CCS are designed to test three different cognitive abilities: recall, application, and analysis. These levels represent an organized way to identify the performance that practitioners will utilize on the job. An explanation of the three cognitive levels is provided here:

Cognitive Level	Purpose	Performance Required
Recall (RE)	Primarily measures memory	Identify terms, specific facts, methods, procedures, basic concepts, basic theories, principles, and processes.
Application (AP)	Measures simple interpretation of limited data	Apply concepts and principles to new situations; recognize relationships among data; apply laws and theories to practical situations; calculate solutions to mathematical problems; interpret charts and translate graphic data; classify items; interpret information.
Analysis (AN)	Measures the application of knowledge to solving a specific problem and the assembly of various elements into a meaningful whole	Select an appropriate solution for responsive action; revise policy, procedure, or plan; evaluate a solution, case scenario, report, or plan; compare solutions, plans, ideas, or aspects of a problem; evaluate information or a situation; perform multiple calculations to arrive at one answer.

CCS Exam Competency Statements

A certification examination is based on an explicit set of competencies. These competencies were determined by job analysis surveys of hospital-based coders. The competencies are subdivided into domains, subdomains, and tasks as shown here. The CCS examination tests only content pertaining to the following competencies.

Domain 1: Health Information Documentation (15%)

1. Interpret health record documentation using knowledge of anatomy, physiology, clinical disease processes, pharmacology, and medical terminology to identify codeable diagnoses and/or procedures.
2. Determine when additional clinical documentation is needed to assign the diagnosis and/or procedure code(s).
3. Consult with physicians and other healthcare providers to obtain further clinical documentation to assist with code assignment.
4. Consult reference materials to facilitate code assignment.
5. Identify patient encounter type.
6. Identify and post charges for healthcare services based on documentation.

Domain 2: Diagnosis Coding (20%)

1. Select the diagnoses that require coding according to current coding and reporting requirements for acute care (inpatient) services.
2. Select the diagnoses that require coding according to current coding and reporting requirements for outpatient services.
3. Interpret conventions, formats, instructional notations, tables and definitions of the classification system to select diagnoses, conditions, problems or other reasons for the encounter that require coding.

4. Sequence diagnoses and other reasons for encounter according to notations and conventions of the classification system and standard data set definitions such as Uniform Hospital Discharge Data Set (UHDDS).

5. Apply the official ICD-9-CM coding guidelines.

Domain 3: Procedure Coding (20%)

1. Select the procedures that require coding according to current coding and reporting requirements for acute care (inpatient) services.

2. Select the procedures that require coding according to current coding and reporting requirements for outpatient services.

3. Interpret conventions, formats, instructional notations, and definitions of the classification system and/or nomenclature to select procedures/services that require coding.

4. Sequence procedures according to notations and conventions of the classification system/nomenclature and standard data set definitions such as UHDDS.

5. Apply the official ICD-9-CM coding guidelines.

6. Apply the official CPT/HCPCS Level II coding guidelines.

Domain 4: Regulatory Guidelines and Reporting Requirements for Acute Care (Inpatient) Service (10%)

1. Select the principal diagnosis, principal procedure, complications, comorbid conditions, other diagnoses and procedures that require coding according to UHDDS definitions and Coding Clinic for ICD-9-CM.

2. Evaluate the impact of code selection on Diagnosis Related Group (DRG) assignment.

3. Verify DRG assignment based on Inpatient Prospective Payment System (IPPS) definitions.

4. Assign the appropriate discharge disposition.

Domain: 5: Regulatory Guidelines and Reporting Requirements for Outpatient Services (10%)

1. Select the reason for encounter, pertinent secondary conditions, primary procedure, and other procedures that require coding according to UHDDS definitions, CPT Assistant, Coding Clinics for ICD-9-CM and HCPCS.

2. Apply Outpatient Prospective Payment System (OPPS) reporting requirements:

    - Modifiers
    - CPT/HCPCS Level II
    - Medical necessity
    - Evaluation and Management code assignment (facility reporting)

Domain 6: Data Quality and Management (8%)

1. Assess the quality of coded data.
2. Educate health care providers regarding reimbursement methodologies, documentation rules and regulations related to coding.
3. Analyze health record documentation for quality and completeness of coding.
4. Review the accuracy of abstracted data elements for data base integrity and claims processing.
5. Review and resolve coding edits such as Correct Coding Initiative (CCI), Medicare Code Editor (MCE) and Outpatient Code Editor (OCE).

Domain 7: Information and Communication Technologies (5%)

1. Use computer to ensure data collection, storage, analysis, and reporting of information.
2. Use common software applications (for example, word processing, spreadsheets, email, etc.) in the execution of work processes.
3. Use specialized software in the completion of HIM processes.

Domain 8: Privacy, Confidentiality, Legal and Ethical Issues (6%)

1. Apply policies and procedures for access and disclosure of personal health information.
2. Apply AHIMA Code of Ethics and the Standards of Ethical Coding.
3. Recognize/report privacy issues/problems.
4. Protect data integrity and validity using software or hardware technology.

Domain 9: Compliance (6%)

1. Participate in the development of institutional coding policies to ensure compliance with official coding rules and guidelines.
2. Evaluate the accuracy and completeness of the patient record as defined by organizational policy and external regulations and standards.
3. Monitor compliance with organization-wide health record documentation and coding guidelines.
4. Recognize/report compliance concerns/findings.

CCS Exam Specifications

Multiple Choice—Part I consists of 60 four-option multiple choice items (50 *scored* items, and 10 *pre-test* items). Pre-test items are unscored items that are included in the examination to assess the item's performance prior to using it for operational use in a future examination. The pre-test items are scrambled randomly throughout the examination and do not count toward the candidate's score.

Medical Record Coding—Part II requires you to code 13 medical records, which contains seven outpatient records (four ambulatory surgery, one emergency room, and two records from Cardiac Cath/Interventional Radiology/Pain Management) and six inpatient records.

- Inpatient diagnoses and procedures are to be coded with ICD-9-CM volumes 1 through 3
- Ambulatory care diagnoses are to be coded with ICD-9-CM volumes 1 and 2; and ambulatory care procedures with CPT.

The total testing time for the exam is four hours. You cannot return to Part I after beginning Part II of the exam.

Time Allotted	Activity
20 minutes	Tutorial (not counted as part of the exam time)
60 minutes	Part I of examination: Multiple Choice section
10 minutes	Mandatory break (not counted as part of the exam time). Retrieve codebooks and collect Part II CCS test booklets from the test center administrator.
180 minutes	Part II of examination: Medical Record Cases

The CCS exam tests accuracy rate and efficiency level of inpatient and outpatient coding. It is important for candidates to pace themselves throughout the exam.

Up to 10 diagnostic and six procedural codes are to be entered on the computer screen in the spaces provided for inpatient records. Up to four ICD-9-CM diagnostic codes and seven CPT procedural codes are to be recorded for ambulatory care records. Medical record coding answers may have fewer codes than the number of spaces provided. Code what is essential, but do not over-code. A penalty applies to inappropriate codes and for a failure to list a required code. Points will be deducted for incorrect codes. Record only the required digits of the codes; do not fill any blank spaces with zeros or other characters. The codes must be typed on the answer sheet in the boxes provided on the computer screen using the keyboard.

For outpatient cases, the scoring is weighted to award more points for appropriately assigning the primary diagnosis. For inpatient cases, the scoring is weighted to award more points for assigning the principal diagnosis; therefore, the principal, not the primary, diagnosis should be assigned. Points are deducted for inappropriate codes.

Follow the procedures (listed earlier) that appear in the Procedures for Coding Part II of the CCS Exam. These procedures will also be supplied with each section of Part II of the exam. Remember that the test will be scored using these procedures. Do not use hospital, regional, or insurance standards that differ from those used in the examination procedures. In order to pass the exam, candidates must meet or exceed the passing scores for both Part I and Part II.

In an effort to improve candidates' testing experience and to provide more space for codebooks, the medical record cases for Part II of the CCS-P exam will be displayed on the computer screen. Navigation will be similar to the multiple choice section of the exam. Candidates will be able to view each case by clicking NEXT, or go back to a previously viewed case by clicking PREVIOUS. Candidates can MARK a case if they want to skip it and return to it at a later time during their exam. The REVIEW button allows you to see an itemized list of the questions. While on the Review screen, questions are displayed as Marked, Completed, or Skipped.

For the CCS exam inpatient and ambulatory coding procedures, please see the Coding Practice section.

What Books to Bring

Please make sure you have the following codebooks when you report to the test center to take your exam.

- 2009 ICD-9-CM Volumes 1 through 3
- 2009 CPT® codebook (published by AMA only)
- Medical dictionary (optional)

For the CCS exam, codebooks are used only in Part II. A medical dictionary may be referenced only in Part II of the exam.

Candidates without the required codebooks will not be permitted to test and will forfeit their application fee. For additional information, please visit http://www.ahima.org/certification.

On Examination Day

The Prometric staff adheres to approved procedures to ensure that the test center meets AHIMA's testing criteria. Please review the following information before the testing date to ensure familiarity with the procedures.

- Plan to arrive at the test center 30 minutes before the scheduled appointment. Candidates arriving at the test center 30 minutes after the scheduled appointment will not be allowed to test and will forfeit the testing fee.
- It is recommended that candidates bring their Authorization to Test (ATT) letter to the test center; however, it is not required to test.
- When arriving at the test center, candidates will be required to present two forms of identification. Please see the following section on identification requirements for a listing of acceptable forms of identification.
- After checking in at the test center, candidates will be directed to the testing area, will have a digital photograph taken, and will be assigned to a testing station. The photograph will be printed on the completion/score report candidates receive after the exam.
- A dry-erase board will be provided for use during the exam.

Identification Requirements

The identification (ID) requirements to be allowed to test include a primary form of ID that contains the candidate's signature and picture, and a secondary form of ID that contains the candidate's signature. The name on the primary and secondary forms of ID should be the same as the name that appears on the testing application.

Acceptable forms of primary ID are valid and non-expired with the candidate's photograph and signature:

- Driver's license
- State ID card
- Government ID card (for example, military ID)
- Passport

Acceptable forms of secondary ID are valid and non-expired with the candidate's printed name and signature:

- Credit or debit card
- Student ID card
- Employee ID card

The following are examples of *unacceptable* forms of ID:

- Expired driver's license or passport
- Social Security card
- Library card
- Marriage certificate
- Voter registration card
- Club membership card
- Public aid card
- Temporary driver's license
- Video club membership card
- Traffic citation (arrest ticket)
- Fishing or hunting license

Without acceptable forms of ID, candidates will not be allowed to test and will forfeit the application fee. Prometric reserves the right to deny a candidate from taking the exam if there is a question in regards to the validity of ID(s).

Test Center Restrictions

To ensure that examination results for all candidates are earned under comparable conditions, it is necessary to maintain a standardized testing environment. Candidates must adhere to the following:

- No reference or study materials may be brought into the examination room. Code books with tabs, handwritten notations, or comments are allowed but must be free of any notes containing coding rules and guidelines from other reference materials (for example, *Coding Clinic*, *CPT® Assistant*, and similar materials). The testing center staff reserves the right to deny code books that contain excessive writing and information that may give the candidate an unfair advantage. Post-It notes and any loose materials are not allowed.
- Documents or notes of any kind may not be removed from the examination room. All computer screens, paper, and written materials are the copyrighted property of Prometric and may not be reproduced in any form.

- Candidates will not be allowed to take anything into the examination room other than those items given to them by the administrator and their identification documents.
- Prohibited items will not be allowed into the examination room. Prohibited items include but are not limited to the following: calculators, pagers, cell phones, electronic digital devices (PDAs, watches), recording or photographic devices, weapons, briefcases, computers or computer bags, and handbags or purses.
- Eating, drinking, and smoking are prohibited in the test center.
- Questions regarding the content of the examination may not be asked of the test center administrator during the exam.

For more CCS examination information, please refer to the 2009 *Certification Candidate Guide* or www.ahima.org/certification.

Introduction

The purpose of this book is to provide practice exercises for the Certified Coding Specialist (CCS) examination through a review of important ICD-9-CM and CPT coding material. A simulation of the CCS exam is also included to improve test performance within the context of the four-hour examination. The content of this book is not intended to predict what will be on the CCS examination because it is not possible for anyone, other than the developers of the examination, to know the content of future examinations.

If you would like to become an AHIMA member, there is an examination discount for both the examination application as well as for AHIMA publication purchases. In addition, you will have access to the AHIMA Communities of Practice (CoP), where there are other resources pertaining to exam topics. The Studying for the CCS CoP is an invaluable community in preparing for the examination. Please visit ahima.org for more information.

Utilizing this review book does not guarantee success in passing the examination; however, it does provide a focused method of preparing for the examination through review, practice, and exam simulation.

Steps for Success

1. Review basic coding principals in basic coding books and then test yourself via the exercises provided in this book.
2. Review relevant *Coding Clinic* articles. Read as many issues of the *Coding Clinic* as possible but be sure to review the most recent five years (2004, 2005, 2006, 2007, 2008) beginning with the most recent articles. As noted, the *Coding Clinic* articles used to develop the 2009 CCS exam end with the fourth quarter of 2008. Knowledge of *Coding Clinic* is crucial for success on the CCS examination. Please be sure to review the most recent *ICD-9-CM Official Guidelines for Coding and Reporting,* which are included in *Coding Clinic.* The national standards for coding practice are provided in *Coding Clinic* and it is therefore the basis for establishing the correct answers related to ICD-9-CM on the CCS exam.
3. Review a CPT educational text and complete exercises for areas in which more skill is needed. Review the Guidelines section of each chapter of the CPT codebook to ensure adequate knowledge of the details of each area.
4. Review the *CPT Assistant* from the most recent issues going backward as far as possible.

5. Complete the introductory sections and practice questions in this book and on CD-ROM.

6. Simulate the actual examination. Use the timing noted below to complete a mock examination *in one sitting.* This book has the ability to have the same number of questions and the same number of inpatient and ambulatory records to be coded as the national examination. You can develop a mock examination based on the types of records you need to be tested on. Follow the exam time frames:

   Part I: 60 minutes for the multiple choice section

   Part II: 180 minutes for coding records

   Try to simulate the actual examination experience as much as possible. This is the experience that successful exam participants find invaluable. It will help you prepare psychologically for the experience of taking a four-hour examination. Make note of any questions.

7. Follow up with study resources and CCS-credentialed professionals to obtain clarification on any items that are unclear. Review any areas of weakness that you identify during the mock examination process.

The codebooks used to develop the 2009 examination are as follows:

- ICD-9-CM codes for fiscal year 2009; these codes were updated on October 1, 2008
- CPT codes for calendar year 2009; these codes were updated on January 1, 2009
- *Coding Clinic* references through the 4th quarter of 2008
- *CPT Assistant* references through December 2008

The 2009 CCS examination is available from June 2009 to May 2010. Please verify this schedule in the current version of the 2009 *Certification Candidate Guide* from AHIMA. For more information on the exam, also refer to the About the CCS Examination section in this book.

Study Resources

ICD-9-CM Coding Resources

Basic ICD-9-CM Coding. 2010. Lou Ann Schraffenberger, MBA, RHIA, CCS, CCS-P. AHIMA product number: AC200509.

Clinical Coding Workout: Practice Exercises for Skill Development, 2009 (with Answers). AHIMA product number: AC201509.

ICD-9-CM Coding Handbook with Answers 2009. Faye Brown. American Hospital Association.

Coding Clinic for ICD-9-CM. American Hospital Association.

ICD-9-CM Official Guidelines for Coding and Reporting. National Center for Vital and Health Statistics (NCHS); available at http://www.cdc.gov/nchs/datawh/ftpserv/ftpicd9/icdguide08.pdf.

HCPCS and CPT Coding Resources

Basic Current Procedural Terminology and HCPCS Coding, 2009. Gail I. Smith, MA, RHIA, CCS-P. AHIMA Product Number: AC200609.

CPT Assistant and *Principles of CPT Coding*. American Medical Association.

2009 HCPCS Codes. HCPCS codes: http://www.cms.hhs.gov/hcpcsreleasecodesets/anhcpcs/List.asp

Regulatory Guidelines, Data Quality, and Compliance Resources

Present on Admission, Second Edition by Gail S. Garrett, RHIT. AHIMA product number: AB121209.

Present on Admission information can be found at www.cms.hhs.gov/HospitalAcqCond.

Severity DRGs and Reimbursement: An MS-DRG Primer by Dr. James S. Kennedy. AHIMA product number: AB215107.

Ingenix 2009 DRG Desk Reference. Ingenix.

Effective Management of Coding Services. Lou Ann Schraffenberger, MBA, RHIA, CCS, CCS-P. Covers a variety of topics such as chargemaster description, quality control issues, compliance, and case-mix analysis. AHIMA product number: AC100007.

MS-DRG Weights. Access to information about the MS-DRG weights for use during 2009: http://www.cms.hhs.gov/acuteinpatientpps/ffd/ItemDetail.asp?ItemID=CMS1213983.

DRG Trees. Information about decision trees, stress management, and other topics can be found at www.mindtools.com/dectree.html. Decision trees form the basis of DRG trees that are found on the national examination. It is important to review this Web site.

APCs and Status Indicator. Access to information about the APCs for use during 2009: http://www.cms.hhs.gov/HospitalOutpatientPPS/06_Annual_Policy_File.asp.

Common medications: www.rxlist.com allows you to check medication and associated diseases.

Health Information Management Compliance: Guidelines for Preventing Fraud and Abuse, Fourth Edition. Sue Bowman, RHIA, CCS. Covers compliance research and trends in an easy-to-understand format. Includes sample auditing and monitoring tools and also provides guidelines for documentation within existing systems, structures for designing a custom compliance program, and what you will need if you are audited. AHIMA product number: AB102107.

Documentation, Information and Communication Technologies and Privacy, Confidentiality, Legal, and Ethical Issues

Health Information Management Technology: An Applied Approach, Second Edition, edited by Merida L. Johns, PhD, RHIA. A valuable resource, useful in all healthcare settings. Students and practicing professionals will find easy-to-understand explanations of the major HIT principles and practical applications to approach real-world situations. AHIMA product number: AB103106.

Health Information Management: Concepts, Principles, and Practice, Third Edition, edited by Kathleen M. LaTour, MA, RHIA, FAHIMA and Shirley Eichenwald Maki, MBA, RHIA, FAHIMA. The most widely used textbook in health information management baccalaureate programs in the country. AHIMA product number: AB103309.

Introduction to Health Information Technology. 2007. Nadinia Davis, MBS, CIA, RHIA, FAHIMA and Melissa LaCour. Elsevier.

Fundamentals of Law for Health Informatics and Health Information Management. Melanie Brodnik, PhD, RHIA , Mary McCain, MPH, RHIA, Laurie Rinehart-Thompson, JD, RHIA, CHP, and Rebecca Reynolds, MHA, RHIA. Offers a practical approach for understanding legal principles impacting HIM. AHIMA product number: AB241807.

HIPAA by Example. Mary C. Thomason, MSA, RHIA, CHPS, CISSP. Offers expert reasoning Privacy Rule applications in various real-life scenarios and clarity on questions outside of those addressed in the Rule itself. Scenarios are based on actual situations, and answers include best practices and reference current state and other laws. AHIMA product number: AB121107.

Electronic Health Records: A Practical Guide for Professionals and Organizations, Fourth Edition. Margret K. Amatayakul, MBA, RHIA, CHPS, CPHIT, CPEHR, FHIMSS. Includes the latest trends and applications in EHRs and offers step-by-step guidelines for developing and implementing EHR strategies. AHIMA product number: AB102608.

Make Plans for CCS Success

In order to develop a good plan of study, it is important to reflect on what you have read so far. Please use a calendar to help determine how much time you have to prepare. Give some thought to what resources you need to help in your preparation as well.

How many hours can you spend per week studying?

____

How many weeks do you have to study before the examination? Take out the weeks when you have personal or family events.

____

____

This table provides information about the passing rate for the CCS exam. Good preparation using the "steps to success" will help to achieve a successful exam experience!

Exam Year	Total Number Taking the Exam	Total Number Passing the Exam	Pass Rate Percentage
2008	1,367	1,068	78%
2007	2,045	936	46%
2006	2,026	1,061	52%
2005	658	301	46%
2004	2,319	1,300	56%
2003	1,901	1,005	53%
2002	1,882	962	51%
2001	1,957	1,403	72%
2000	1,856	1,142	62%
1999	1,498	1,025	68%
1998	1,188	812	68%

Sources: E-mail correspondence from AHIMA staff, 2009. *Journal of the AHIMA.*

Self-Evaluation Notes

Each person who studies for the CCS exam has a different skill set. One of the goals for using this book is to determine your areas of weakness. Strategies can then be developed to make weak areas stronger. Take a few minutes to complete this short self-evaluation so that your specific needs can be addressed. Use this self-evaluation to help gather resources before working through the remainder of this book.

I need more practice in these areas:

1. ______________________________

2. ______________________________

3. ______________________________

I can strengthen these areas by:

1. ______________________________

2. ______________________________

3. ______________________________

I need these resources to help me:

1. ______________________________

2. ______________________________

3. ______________________________

Coding Challenges

The following is an outline of potentially challenging coding issues. If possible, obtain the reference materials listed here and utilize them in your study process. In accordance with the study calendar developed in this book, spend the specified hours per week studying the coding materials so that your areas of weakness are addressed. Planning a schedule and obtaining materials that address your weaknesses will enable you to achieve your goals. Many people find that meeting with a small study group each week in person can help you stay on track. In addition to in-person study group support, there is an AHIMA Community of Practice, Studying for the CCS, which can provide online assistance and resources. As you review the different areas of content, identify any weaknesses that you need to focus on for improvement.

In order to do well on the multiple choice section of this book, reference material related to the exam content will need to be memorized. It is not possible to memorize everything, so developing a study strategy is important. A core strategic approach should include reading the About the CCS Examination section to fully understand the examination contents and what should be coded, determining weak areas and studying to improve those areas, and focusing on clinical scenarios and reimbursement topics that would apply to the average hospital.

Keep in mind that during the CCS exam you are only allowed to use your codebooks during part II. Furthermore, materials in codebooks must be permanently affixed inside your codebooks. (Refer to the 2009 *Certification Candidate Guide.*) Remember too that you will need to gain speed using the codebooks because the encoder is not used to assign codes during the examination. In order to hone this skill, practice coding exercises by timing yourself to evaluate your speed and accuracy using only actual codebooks.

The following are highlights to remember:

- Because national coding guidelines and references are used for the CCS examination, evaluate your hospital guidelines to identify any difference between the two. Be sure to code according to national guidelines during the CCS examination.
- Recent issues addressed in *Coding Clinic* and *CPT Assistant* are important to know. Begin your review of *Coding Clinic* and *CPT Assistant* from the most recent to the oldest issues. Identify areas that are confusing or have been revised over time. Make sure you understand the most recent decision regarding any particular coding issue.
- Knowledge of MS-DRGs and APCs is very important. Which DRGs will be affected by major comorbidities or complications (MCCs) and complications or comorbidities (CCs) is key information. You should have a general idea about common MS-DRGs

for the average hospital in the United States and the reimbursement methodology of APCs. For example, what the status indicators mean and how to assign evaluation and management (E/M) levels if given a template.

- An understanding of accurate principal assignment is key as well. It is essential to know the disease processes that underlie ethical coding. Much of this knowledge is based in *Coding Clinic* reference material and the Uniform Hospital Discharge Data Set (UHDDS).
- Generally, cases on the examination reflect common cases that a coder in an average hospital would code. Determine if you have a knowledge deficit in any common coding areas because your facility does not treat that type of patient. For example, some facilities do not provide services for newborns, deliveries, heart catheterization, and coronary artery bypass grafts (CABGs), or neonatal intensive care. If you work in such a facility, you will need to strategize how to gather expertise in these areas. One way to gain expertise is to review the coding exercises in the basic coding book and to use the encoder to determine the MS-DRGs associated with the exercises.
- Remember that national coding principles are emphasized on the CCS examination. A review of the last two years of the *Journal of the American Health Information Management Association* is a worthwhile endeavor. Be mindful of such topics as future nomenclatures such as ICD-10, CPT-5, and the Health Insurance Portability and Accountability Act (HIPAA). Also, keep in mind that sometimes coders get into habits that may subtly deviate from coding guidelines. Be on alert and identify any of these habits in order to correct them.

ICD-9-CM Review

The following is an outline of some of the more important areas to know.

Infectious Disease

Review the most recent guidelines regarding sepsis (038.x + SIRS code) versus septicemia (038.x). They require that a code from 038 be used followed by 995.91. If septic shock is also documented, 995.92 and 785.52 should be assigned.

Diabetes

- Review the definition of fifth digits in this category.
- Understand the difference between type I and type II diabetes and the pathophysiology of both types.

Respiratory

- Remember to use the code for the specific type of pneumonia if the cause of the pneumonia is documented in the medical record by the provider.
- Know the criteria for recognizing gram-negative and other specific types of pneumonia when documented in the medical record.

- Review the various types of chronic obstructive pulmonary disease (COPD) and how the acute exacerbation of each is coded. Know the criteria for coding asthma with status asthmaticus as specified in *Coding Clinic* and code only when documented in the record.
- Review the criteria for coding respiratory failure and when it may be sequenced first.

Procedures

- Understand how procedures, sometimes performed at the patient's bedside, affect the MS-DRG assignment. Some examples are transbronchial biopsies, ventilator usage, excisional debridement, and tracheostomies.
- Be careful to assign debridement codes appropriately. Do not code an excisional debridement unless there is documentation in the record reflecting that an excisional debridement was performed.

Gastrointestinal

- Use a combination code whenever available that incorporates a hemorrhage and the specific disorder. Use the 578.x category as an additional code when no combination code has been created or when the cause of the hemorrhage is unknown.
- Understand the difference between a direct (no path report) versus an indirect hernia (path report will show a hernia sac) and how to code them.

Delivery and Pregnancy

- Understand the definition of fifth digits and when to use them. Remember that the fifth digit of 4 is only used for a postpartum complication not in the same episode of the delivery. If you work at a facility that does not perform deliveries, use the review exercises in another coding text to improve your knowledge in this area.
- Memorize the definition of a normal delivery and know the parameters for using the 650 code.
- Recognize that, at a minimum, delivery charts must have the following types of codes: delivery diagnosis code (600 code), outcome of delivery (V2x.xx), and procedure code (73.59 if no other procedure performed).
- Remember that medical conditions associated with pregnancy, delivery, and puerperium require both a 6XX code as well as a disease code. For example, postpartum anemia is coded as 648.22 and 285.9.

Ectopic Pregnancy and Miscarriages

- Understand the definition of fifth digits and when to use them.
- Understand how to code complications of ectopic pregnancy and abortions during the admission for treatment of the ectopic pregnancy or abortion. Review the inclusion notes for 639.x category in the ICD tabular (the section ordered by number) and know when to use it.

Anemia

- Review the anemia coding. In particular, there are new anemia codes for anemia in chronic illness. Also, blood loss anemia is a commonly associated condition with chronic bleeding and acute bleeding. Be sure to know when to code acute versus chronic blood loss anemia. It is also important to review national guidelines regarding postoperative anemia.

Cardiovascular Conditions

- Remember to specify the location of the myocardial infarction and any comorbidities that will affect the DRG assignment such as arrhythmias, heart failure, hypotension, and so on.
- Review and understand sequencing issues pertaining to ASHD and unstable angina in *Coding Clinic.*
- Review the coding of cerebral infarctions and sequelae such as aphasia and hemiplegia.
- Review coding cardiac procedures such as cardiac catheterizations and bypass surgery. If you do not have exposure to this type of chart, try to practice coding these issues using a coding exercise book.

Neoplasms

- Review the definitions of the categories in the table.
    - The primary site is where the cancer arises.
    - A secondary neoplasm is present whenever the neoplasm leaves the organ of origin (where it began). This can occur when the neoplasm travels through the blood and/or the lymphatic system or via direct growth (direct extension) into another adjacent tissue.
- Remember that looking up the morphology type can lead you to the primary (for example, cell carcinoma arises in the kidney).
- Review the suggested steps in *ICD-9-CM Coding Handbook with Answers,* which are synopsized as follows:
    - Look up the morphology and code the primary site if given.
    - If no primary site code is indicated by the morphology type, the neoplasm table must be used.
    - Use the following list if the term "metastatic" is used ambiguously. Assume the following are secondary sites: bone, brain, diaphragm, heart, liver, lymph nodes, mediastium, meninges, peritoneum, pleura, retroperitoneum, spinal cord, and sites from 195 category.

Injuries and Burns

- Review the difference between traumatic versus pathological fractures.
- Make sure the most extensive wound is coded and all injured internal organs are coded.

- Review the fifth digits related to intracranial injury, and make sure the appropriate code is used.
- Remember that if burns are located in the same body area, use only the degree of greatest severity. For example, if there are second- and third-degree burns of the forearm, only the third-degree burn of the forearm is coded.

Drugs

- Review the difference between abuse and addiction and the fifth digits associated with them. Also review the coding of procedures associated with this area.
- Review the definition of adverse effect. The following terms indicate an adverse effect of a drug:
    - Allergic reaction
    - Cumulative effect
    - Hypersensitivity
    - Idiosyncratic reaction
    - Paradoxical reaction
    - Synergistic
- Review the definition of poisoning. The following are classified as poisonings when:
    - The drug is administered, taken, or prescribed incorrectly, for example, if an overdose of medication occurs
    - Alcohol is used in conjunction with a drug
    - Street drugs are taken resulting in an overdose or taken in addition to prescribed or over-the-counter (OTC) drugs
    - OTCs are taken with prescriptions
    - Two OTC drugs are used together

Complications

- Review this section of the ICD-9-CM codebook to refresh your memory about how these codes are found. Review the alphabetic and tabular indices and what is contained within each category.
- The best way to review this area is to go through the tabular index (the section ordered by number).
- The first area in the tabular contains the three major groupings associated with devices and complications (in the Complications chapter):
    - Mechanical Complications (996.0–996.59)
    - Infection/Inflammation Due to Devices (996.6–996.69)
    - Other Complications (996.7–996.79)

- Review the general complications in the 997 and 998 categories. Remember that a second code is required because of the directions given under the main heading of 997. A second code should also be used with 998 to denote the specific manifestation, if the code is not specific to the exact type of complication. For example, if a patient has intraoperative atrial fibrillation, use 997.1 and 427.31; and if a patient has postoperative septicemia, use 998.59 and 038.9.
- Review the 999 category as well. Issues such as phlebitis due to IV are listed here.
- Complications that occur only in specific body sites are classified in that chapter of the ICD-9-CM codebook. For example, postoperative pulmonary embolism (415.11) is found in Chapter 8, "Respiratory System." Complications of abortion, pregnancy, labor, or delivery are classified to Chapter 11.

Perinatal Conditions

- Use the V code (V3x.xx) as principal when the admission is for the birth of the infant. Do not use V3x.xx if the admission is not for birth (for example, the patient is transferred).
- Use other perinatal conditions as appropriate such as birth trauma, prematurity, jaundice, and so on when documented in the record.

MS-DRGs/Case Mix

If you do not code inpatient records on a routine basis, it is important to obtain a list of MS-DRGs from www.cms.hhs.gov/home/medicare.asp (search for DRG relative weights). If you can, put some of the exercises or cases in this book in the MS-DRG grouper so you can familiarize yourself with common MS-DRGs. Switch the principal diagnosis and note how the MS-DRG changes. This will help familiarize you with MS-DRGs. Also note which MS-DRGs are affected by MCCs.

Review the MS-DRG weights of the most common MS-DRGs that would occur in the average hospital in the United States. The following is a list, which is by no means is all inclusive, of some common clinical scenarios that may form the basis of further study.

Pneumonia
Congestive Heart Failure
Cholecystitis and Cholecystectomy
Malignant Neoplasms with Associated Treatments
  Lung
  Breast
  Prostate
  Colon
Fracture of Femur with Associated Treatments
  Total Hip Replacement
  Open Reduction with Internal Fixation
Septicemia
Gastrointestinal Hemorrhage

COPD with Exacerbation
Respiratory Failure
Deliveries
Newborns
Anemia

Case mix (CM) is defined as the volume and type of cases. If all of the weights of all the MS-DRGs were added together, this would provide the case mix for a given patient population. The *case mix index* (CMI) is defined as the average case. To calculate the CMI, you must add all the weights together and divide by the number of patients.

Review the common MS-DRGs that cannot be optimized unless a procedure is found or the principal diagnosis is changed (for example, DRG 127, 416, and 294). Try to find more.

Use a grouper that you have access to in your work or academic institution or visit www.irp.com to use a free DRG grouper. *Disclaimer: This software application may contain errors and is not endorsed or developed by the author or AHIMA.*

The following exercises are meant to help you learn more about case mix analysis and increase your knowledge of MS-DRGs. In actual coding practice, it would only be appropriate to switch the principal diagnoses if the clinical information conformed to UHDDS guidelines that supported a change in principal diagnosis. Try these exercises:

1. A 22-month-old child has pyelonephritis (590.80) and dehydration (276.51) and both are equally treated. Which MS-DRG will have the highest weight?
2. If a 65-year-old patient has pneumonia (486) and congestive heart failure (428.0), which DRG will have a higher weight?
3. If a 70-year-old patient has pneumonia due to *Escherichia coli* (482.82) and an acute exacerbation of COPD (491.21), which DRG will have a higher weight?
4. Case Mix (CM) and Case Mix Index (CMI) Calculations: The CM is all of the weights added together. The CMI is the average weight of all the cases in a given dataset or period of time. What is the case mix and CMI for these cases using the highest paying MS-DRGs?

Answers

1. 590.80 has a weight of .0.7581, whereas 276.51 has a weight of 0.682. In this case the pyelonephritis used as principal results in a higher-paying MS-DRG.
2. 486 has a weight of 0.7316, whereas 428.0 has a weight of 1.4601. The CHF MS-DRG has a higher weight.
3. 482.82 has a weight of 1.4983, whereas 491.21 has a weight of 1.303. The pneumonia DRG has a higher weight.
4. CM = 0.7581 + 1.4601 + 1.4983 = 3.7165, CMI = 3.7165 / 3 = 1.239

CPT Review

Review the beginning of each section in the CPT codebook for instructions about definitions and other information pertinent to assigning the correct code. The following are points to review:

Integumentary (Skin)

- Review the section on lacerations (repair) in the CPT book regarding when to add the lengths together and when to use an addition code for closure of the wound.
- Remember that grafts are measured in square centimeters (this is different from lacerations).
- Review the use of codes involved in excision, destruction, or other methods of removing lesions in the Malignant, Benign, Skin Tags, Other Lesions section.

Endoscopies

- In general, the alphabetical index will provide a range of codes for a given procedure. Some of these are open procedures. Make sure you look up each code before assigning it.
- There is a difference between "brushings and washings" and a biopsy in CPT.
    - Review the definitions of upper and lower gastrointestinal (GI) endoscopies in CPT
    - Upper gastrointestinal endoscopy
    - Proctosigmoidoscopy
    - Sigmoidoscopy
    - Colonoscopy
    - Review the laparoscopy section of CPT
    - Review the definitions of the sinus procedures
    - Review the definitions under bronchoscopies. Remember that a bilateral bronchoscopy is coded twice or with a modifier –50.

Musculoskeletal

- Review the terminology differences between ICD and CPT related to the treatment of fractures. For example, "manipulation" is the same in CPT as "reduction" in ICD-9.
- Understand the medical terminology, approaches, notes, and inclusions for knee repairs.

Outpatient Prospective Payment System

- The Outpatient Prospective Payment System (OPPS) began to be used for Medicare in August 2000. This system uses the ambulatory payment classifications (APCs) for reimbursement for hospital-based outpatient services such as outpatient surgery, emergency department visits, outpatient clinic visits, and outpatient ancillary tests. Some highlights of this system are listed here:

- APCs are similar to MS-DRGs in that they are both prospective payment methodologies and both have relative weights.
- APCs are different from MS-DRGs because outpatients can have multiple APCs for a given encounter, whereas an inpatient can have only one MS-DRG.
- APCs are generated for many services, such as x-rays, medical tests, clinic or emergency visits, surgical procedures, devices, drugs and biologicals, and partial hospitalizations.
- The billing number is the connecting identifier for a given patient's encounter that results in multiple APCs.
- Status indicators denote what type of service was provided and assist in determining the payment. Status indicators include: X, ancillary; V, clinic or emergency department visit; T, significant procedure that is discounted when other T procedures are provided (the first procedure is paid at a rate of 100 percent whereas the second and those thereafter are paid at 50 percent); S, significant procedure that is paid at 100 percent and is not discounted; P, partial hospitalization; H, devices; G/J, drugs/biologicals; K, non-pass-through drugs/biologicals. Please visit the CMS Web page as noted in the reference section of the book for more information.
- CPT (numeric) and HCPCS (alphanumeric) modifiers approved for hospital outpatient are listed on the CPT codebook inside cover; –25, –27,–50, –52, –58, –59, –73, –74, –76, –77, –78, –79, –91, –LT, –RT, –CA, –E1, –E2, –E3, –E4, –FA, –F1, –F2, –F3, –F4, –F5, –F6, –F7, –F8, –F9, –GA, –GG, –GH, –LC, –LD, –QM, –QN, –RC, –TA, –T1, –T2, –T3, –T4, –T5, –T6, –T7, –T8, –T9.
- The following illustration is a hypothetical example of one patient's APCs for a given encounter in the emergency department.

Billing Number	Status Indicator	CPT/HCPC	APC	Amount
789321	Q	99284–25	0615	$315.51
789321	T	25500	0043	$197.50
789321	X	72050	0261	$73.69
789321	S	72128	0332	$191.78
789321	S	70450	0332	$191.78
				Reimbursement Total = $970.26

You should review *Coding Clinic* and *CPT Assistant* with three goals in mind.

- Review the past three to five years of both references to prepare for the multiple choice and coding sections of the examination. Review at least the past three years of every issue in both references beginning with the most recent issue and reading backward (for instance read 4th Quarter 2008, then 3rd Quarter 2008). This will allow you to know when changes have occurred and what the most recent requirements are.

- Review as many topics that pertain to common inpatient and outpatient diagnoses and procedures for services that the average hospital would provide. Be sure to read the official coding guidelines beginning with the most recent version.
- Bolster knowledge in your areas of weakness that you have identified. The references for the 2009 CCS examination will stop at the end of 2008.

Coding Clinic

Review relevant areas of common diagnoses and MS-DRGs to prepare for the multiple-choice section. In addition to the targeted review of topics, also review each issue of *Coding Clinic* for the past three years beginning with the most recent issue. You should know the most recent guidelines and any previous guidelines that have been changed.

CPT Assistant

Review relevant areas to common outpatient procedures. In addition to the targeted review listed here, also review each issue for the past three years.

Review of CCS Annual Self-Assessment for Credential Maintenance Questions

2007

Content Area	Topic	Reference
ICD-9-CM Diagnosis Coding	1. Myeloproliferative disorders	*CC 4th Quarter 2006*, 64
ICD-9-CM Diagnosis Coding	2. Injuries following an accident	*CC 1st Quarter 2006*, 9
ICD-9-CM Diagnosis Coding	3. Chronic hepatitis C infection	*CC 2nd Quarter 2006*, 13
ICD-9-CM Diagnosis Coding	4. Heart failure with heart valve disorders	*CC 3rd Quarter 2006*, 7
Regulatory Inpatient	5. SIRS, sepsis and severe sepsis	11/15/06 *ICD-9-CM Official Coding Guidelines*, Section I.C.1.b
Health Information Documentation	6. Coding metastatic sites from pathology reports	*CC 1st Quarter 2006*, 8
ICD-9-CM Diagnosis Coding	7. Coding "mass" of a site not listed in the diagnostic index	*CC 1st Quarter 2006*, 4
ICD-9-CM Diagnosis Coding	8. Ventilator-associated pneumonia	*CC 2nd Quarter 2006*, 25
ICD-9-CM Diagnosis Coding	9. Acute exacerbation of COPD, acute bronchitis, and acute exacerbation of asthma	*CC 3rd Quarter 2006*, 20
ICD-9-CM Procedure Coding	10. Subcutaneous treatment of prostate cancer	*CC 1st Quarter 2006*, 10
ICD-9-CM Procedure Coding	11. Correct ICD-9-CM procedure codes for suture of an artery after ECMO	*CC 3rd Quarter 2006*, 9

Content Area	Topic	Reference
ICD-9-CM Procedure Coding	12. Excisional débridement with skin substitute	*CC 3rd Quarter 2006*, 19
ICD-9-CM Procedure Coding	13. Repeat C-section, multiple adhesions, and vacuum usage	*CC 2nd Quarter 2006*, 5
CPT	14. Code for replacement of double-J ureteral stent	*CPT Assistant,* September 2006, 2
CPT	15. Coding rules for 25600 and 25650	*2007 CPT Codebook*, 98
CPT	16. Laser treatments for prostate	*CPT Assistant,* November 2006, 21
CPT	17. Salivary gland biopsy	*CPT Changes 2007—An Insider's View,* 116
CPT	18. Modified Maze procedure	*CPT Changes 2007—An Insider's View,* 75–77
CPT	19. Laparoscopic implantation of neurostimulator electrodes in stomach	*CPT Changes 2007—An Insider's View,* 116–117
CPT	20. Open reduction of distal radial intra-articular fracture with internal fixation	*CPT Changes 2007—An Insider's View,* 63
CPT	21. Repair of the brachial and ulnar nerves using synthetic nerve tubes	*CPT Changes 2007—An Insider's View,* 154
HCPCS	22. G codes	http://a257.g.akamaitech.net/7/257/2422/01jan20061800/edocket.access.gpo.gov/2006/pdf/06
Regulatory Inpatient	23. POA Guidelines	11/15/06 *ICD-9-CM Official Coding Guidelines*, Appendix I, 90
Regulatory Outpatient	24. Medically Unlikely Edits	http://cms.hhs.gov/transmittals/downloads/R178PI.pdf
Health Information Documentation	25. Diagnoses related to a colon resection	*CC 1st Quarter 2006*, 7–8

2008

Content Area	Topic	Reference
ICD-9-CM Diagnosis Coding	1. PICC-associated infection	*CC 4th Quarter 2007*, 96–97
Regulatory Inpatient	2. Pain codes	*Official Coding Guidelines* effective 10/1/07 Section I.C.6.a
ICD-9-CM Diagnosis Coding	3. Gastric Ulcer and Diverticulitis	*CC 2nd Quarter 2007*, 11
ICD-9-CM Diagnosis Coding	4. Chest pain with likely gastrointestinal-type disorder	*CC 1st Quarter 2007*, 19
ICD-9-CM Diagnosis Coding	5. Postoperative anemia due to acute blood loss	*CC 1st Quarter*, 19
Health Information Documentation	6. Documentation of chronic secondary conditions	*CC 3rd Quarter 2007*, 13
Regulatory Inpatient	7. Principal Diagnosis for control of pain due to malignancy	*CC 2nd Quarter 2007*, 13
Data Quality and Management	8. Non-Hodgkins lymphomas	*CC 4th Quarter 2007*, 65
ICD-9-CM Procedure Coding	9. Automatic external defibrillator	*CC 1st Quarter 2007*, 17–18
ICD-9-CM Procedure Coding	10. Arteriovenous fistula creation	*CC 1st Quarter 2007*, 18
ICD-9-CM Procedure Coding	11. Insertion facet replacement device	*CC 4th Quarter 2007*, 116–120
ICD-9-CM Procedure Coding	12. Insertion Tulip filter	*CC 2nd Quarter 2007*, 4
ICD-9-CM Procedure Coding	13. Thoracoscopic lobectomy	*CC 4th Quarter 2007*, 109–113
CPT	14. Detection of MRSA by amplified probe	*CPT Assistant,* August 2007, 7
CPT	15. Excision of malignant lesion with intermediate or complex closure	*CPT 2008 Professional Edition*, 55
CPT	16. New tube for colonic tube	*CPT 2008 Professional Edition*, 218
CPT	17. Additional code for placement of nasogastric tube to insufflate the stomach	*CPT Changes 2008—An Insider's View,* 137
CPT	18. Cryoablation of renal tumors	*CPT 2008 Professional Edition*, 226
CPT	19. Techniques for tissue ablation, disruption, and reconstruction	*CPT 2008 Professional Edition*, 146
CPT	20. Arthroscopy of subtalar joint with removal of loose body	*CPT 2008 Professional Edition*, 130
CPT	21.Limited hepatic magnetic resonance imaging	*CPT Assistant,* November 2007, 9
Regulatory Outpatient	22. Guidelines for pediatric patient transport	*CPT 2008 Professional Edition*, 18

Content Area	Topic	Reference
Data Quality and Management	23. Transient Ischemic Attacks Defined	CC 1st Quarter 2007, 24
Regulatory Inpatient	24. Postoperative pain codes	*Official Coding Guidelines* effective 10/1/07 Chapter 6 number 3, 28
Regulatory Outpatient	25. Type of fracture correlated to type of treatment	*CPT Assistant,* October 2007, 7–13

HIM professionals who have the CCS credential must undertake a self-assessment each year to maintain their credential. If you can obtain these self-assessments from a coworker or friend, they will be a good resource from which to study for the exam.

CCS Domain	Introduction and Coding Challenges	CCS Examination Simulation Multiple Choice Questions
1. Health Information Documentation	Health Information Documentation, Information and Communication Technologies, and Privacy, Confidentiality, Legal and Ethical Issues	5, 8, 27, 29, 33, 42, 57, 60
2. Diagnosis Coding	ICD-9-CM Coding Resources	1, 4, 13, 22, 24, 37, 39, 41, 46, 49, 54, 55, 56
3. Procedure Coding	HCPCS and CPT Resources	1, 2, 3, 4, 9, 16, 22, 25, 28, 30, 32, 34, 35, 52
4. Regulatory Inpatient	Regulatory Guidelines, Data Quality, and Compliance Resources	14, 15, 17, 21, 23, 26, 38, 44, 47, 50, 59
5. Regulatory Outpatient	Regulatory Guidelines, Data Quality, and Compliance Resources	18, 19, 20, 36, 45
6. Data Quality and Management	Regulatory Guidelines, Data Quality, and Compliance Resources	40, 10, 11, 12
7. Information and Communication Technologies	Health Information Documentation, Information and Communication Technologies, and Privacy, Confidentiality, Legal and Ethical Issues	58, 48, 43
8. Privacy, Confidentiality, Legal, and Ethical Issues	Health Information Documentation, Information and Communication Technologies, and Privacy, Confidentiality, Legal and Ethical Issues	31, 51, 53
9. Compliance	Regulatory Guidelines, Data Quality, and Compliance Resources	6, 7, 2

Common Diseases and Disorders with Associated Drugs

This is *not* a comprehensive list of conditions and drugs that may occur. It is simply a short summary of common conditions and associated medications that may be found in medical records. For more information about medications and diseases, visit www.rxlist.com.

AIDS—An immunodeficiency syndrome caused by the human immunodeficiency virus (HIV). This disorder is associated with opportunistic infections, malignancies, and neurologic disease.
Medications: NRTIs-Nucleoside Reverse Transcriptase Inhibitors (Retrovir, AZT, Videx, ddl, Hivid, ddC, Zeril, d4tT, Epivir, 3TC); NRTIs-Nonnucleoside Reverse Transcriptase Inhibitors (Viramunde, Sustiva); Protease Inhibitors; (Invirase, Saquinavir, Crixovan, Indinavir, Kaletra, Lipinavir, Ritinavir).

Allergies—A hypersensitivity to a substance that does not normally cause a reaction.
Medications: antihistamines such as Claritin, Phenergan, Allegra, Zyrtec. The most common antihistamine for allergic reaction is diphenhydramine (Benadryl).

Anemia—A reduction in the number of circulating red blood cells or a reduction in the amount of hemoglobin in each red blood cell.
Medications: iron supplements, ferrous sulfate (Feosol), ferrous fumarate (Femiron), ferrous gluponate (Fergon); B12 (Cyanocobalamin); hematopoietic agents (Procrit, Epogen, Neupogen).

Angina Pectoris—Severe pain associated with constriction in blood vessels to the heart with pain radiating to the left arm, abdomen, back, or jaw.
Medications: verapamil (Verelan, Calan SR); diltiazem (Cardizem CD, Dilacor); nifedipine (Adalat, Procardia); nitrates (Isordil, Imdur, ISMO); NTG-nitroglycerin (Nitroquick, Nitrodur); atenolom (Tenormin).

Anxiety—A mental disorder that manifests as fear, worry, or dread that is not related to a specific event or set of objects.
Medications: lorazepam (Ativan); alprazolam (Xanax); diazepam (Valium); paroxetine (Paxil); buspirone (Buspar).

Arrhythmia—Irregularities in the force or rhythm of the heart such as atrial fibrillation, tachycardia, bradycardia, or cardiac arrest.
Medications: verapamil (Calan SR, Verelan); digoxin (Lanoxin); quinidine (Quinaglute, Quinidex); amiodarone (Cordarone).

Arthritis—Inflammation of the joints. There are three major types of arthritis: osteoarthritis, rheumatoid arthritis, and gout.
Medications: ibuprofen (Advil, Motrin); hydrocortisone; Lodine; naproxen (Naprosyn; Oruvail; prednisone (Deltasone); Relafen; Voltaren; Medrol; Daypro; Celebrex.

Asthma—A spasm of the bronchial tubes or swelling of the mucous membrane.
Medications: Albuterol (Proventil, Ventolin); theophylline; TheoDur; Serevent; Xopenea; Azmocort; Atroverit.

Bipolar Disorder—A mental disorder in which both mania and depression occur.
Medications: lithium; Lithobid; Eskalith; Zyprexa.

Chronic Obstructive Pulmonary Disease (COPD)—A group of disorders that decrease the ability of the lungs to provide ventilation to the body. Some forms of COPD include: chronic obstructive asthma, chronic obstructive bronchitis, emphysema, bronchiectasis, and combinations of the aforementioned disorders.
Medications: Prednisone, albuterol (Proventil, Ventolin); Serevent; Alupent; Atrovent.

Congestive Heart Failure—The inability of the heart to pump the blood through the body adequately, resulting in edema in the extremities.
Medications: Bumex; Dyazide; furosemide (Lasix); HCTZ-hydrochlorothiazide; Lozol; digoxin (Lanoxin).

Dehydration—The loss of body fluid. This may be associated with severe nausea and vomiting, diarrhea, high fever, and urinary tract infections.
Medications: intravenous fluids, oral fluids; Pedialyte; Infalyte; Gatorade; Sportade.

Depression—A mental disorder in which there is loss of interest in usually pleasurable pursuits.
Medications: amitriptyline hydrochloride (Elavil); Celexa; nortriptyline hydrochloride (Pamelor); Paxil; Prozac; trazodone hydrochloride (Desyrel); Zoloft.

Diabetes Mellitus—A disorder in which there is inadequate production or utilization of insulin. There are two types: Type I (the body does not produce or does not produce enough endogenous insulin) and Type II (the cells of the body do not utilize the endogenous insulin properly).
Medications: glyburide (DiaBeta, Glynase Prestab, Micronase); Glucophage, Glucotrol; insulin (Humulin, Humalog, Novolin), Lantus.

Diverticulitis—An infection of the diverticula that causes inflammation.
Medications: antibiotics: ampicillin; gentamicin; tetracycline; cephalosporins (Mefoxin, Rocephin, Fortaz).

Diverticulosis—Formation of diverticula in the large intestine that can bleed or become infected/inflamed.
Medications: High-fiber diet.

Fever—An elevated temperature.
Medications: acetaminophen (Tylenol); aspirin; ibuprofen (Motrin, Advil, Nuprin).

Gastrointestinal ulcers—A lesion in the mucosal membrane of the gastrointestinal tract that may cause bleeding or perforation. When a perforation occurs, the bacteria in the gastrointestinal tract may spill into the adjacent body cavity, causing peritonitis.
Medications: (Axid; Nexium; Pepcid; Prilosec; Tagamet; Zantac).

Hyperlipidemia—An excessive amount of lipids (fat) in the blood.
Medications: gemfibrozil (Lopid, Mevacor, Pravachol, Zocor, Lipitor).

Hypertension—Blood pressure that is persistently higher than normal. Malignant hypertension is characterized by severe vascular and other internal organ damage.
Medications: Altace; atenolol (Tenormin); Accupril; Capoten; Cardura; Coreg; Corgard; DynaCirc; enalapril (Vasotec); Hytrin; Lotensin; metropolol (Lopressor); Norvasc; Prinivil; Zestril.

Hypokalemia—Potassium depletion in the blood.
Medications: potassium chloride (K-Dur, K-Lyte, Micro-K, Klor-Con, K-Tab, Kaon, K-Lor).

Hypotension—Persistently lower-than-normal blood pressure. There are two common forms of hypotension: orthostatic, and that due to other disorders such as anemia, trauma, hemorrhage, and fever.
Medications: volume expansion by increasing salt (NaCl); fludrocortisone acetate (Florinef Acetate); ephedrine.

Hypothyroid—A decreased amount of thyroid secretion.
Medications: Levoxyl; Synthroid; thyroid; Levothroid; Cytomel.

Impotence—Inability to maintain or achieve erection. This can occur because of an organic cause: following a radical prostatectomy, due to diabetes or alcohol abuse, or due to medications. Psychological reasons can also be a cause of this disorder.
Medications: Viagra; alprastadil (Muse, Edex, Caverject).

Infection—The result of an invasion of a pathogenic agent such as a virus or a bacterium. Infectious organisms include: bacteria (such as streptococci, staphylococci, spirochetes), viruses, fungi, and protozoa.
Medications: antibiotics; amoxicillin trihydrate (Amoxil); ampicillin; Augmentin; Bactroban; Beepen-VK; Biaxin; Ceclor; Ceftin; Cefzil; cephalexin; Cipro; Claforan; Cotrim; doxycycline; Duricef; erythromycin (E.E.S.,E-Mycin 333, Erythrcin, EryTab); Floxin; Fortaz; Lorabid; Macrobid; neomycin and polymixin; Penicillin VK; Pen-Vee K; Peridex; Principen; Rocephine; Suprax; tetracycline; Trimox; Vantin; Veetids; Zithromax; antifungals; Diflucan; Lotrisone; Nizoral; nystatin; antivirals; amvir; Valtrex; metronidazole; Zovirax.

Malignant neoplasms—The uncontrolled growth of cells and the dispersion of malignant cells through the blood, the lymph system, or by direct extension to tissue adjacent to the tumor.
Medications: chemotherapy; 5-Fluorovracil; chlorambucil; cisplatin (Platinol); Cytoxan; doxorubicin (Adriamycin); Flutamide, megestrol acetate (Megace), MTX-methotrexate; prednisone; Taxol; Taxotere; vinblastine (Velban); vincristine (Oncovin); hormonal therapy; Arimidex; goserelin (Zoladex); Lupron; Proscar; Tamoxifen; biological response modifiers; Herceptin; Intron; Proleukin, IL-2; Roferon.

Pneumonia or Pneumonitis—An infection or inflammation of the lungs. There are multiple causes such as infectious agents (bacterial or virus), aspiration of secretions or food, inhalation of fumes, or radiation.
Medications: See *infections.*

Septicemia—A systemic infection usually manifesting in pathogenic organisms or accumulation of their toxins in the bloodstream.
Medications: See *infections.*

Thrombophlebitis—Inflammation of a vein. This condition leaves the patient at risk for embolisms.
Medication: warfarin sodium (Coumadin); heparin.

Schizophrenia—A group of disorders characterized by disordered thinking, effect, and behavior.
Medications: haloperidol (Haldol); chlorpromazine (Thorazine); thioridazine (Mellaril); fluphenazine (Prolixin); Serentil; Seroquel; Clozaril; Zyprexa.

Seizure—Involuntary muscular contractions and relaxations.
Medications: Depakote; Dilantin; Klonopin; Neurontin; phenobarbital; Tegretol; diazepam (Valium); Topamax.

Coding Practice

The questions in this section are based on principles from basic coding texts. Identify problems as you work through these questions, and then review the corresponding chapter(s) identified in one of the texts.

Exam Coding Procedures

Ambulatory Care Coding

1. Apply ICD-9-CM instructional notations and conventions and current approved "Basic Coding Guidelines for Outpatient Services" and "Diagnostic Coding and Reporting Requirements for Physician Billing" (*Coding Clinic for ICD-9-CM,* 4th Quarter 1995 and 1996) to select diagnoses, conditions, problems, or other reasons for care that require ICD-9-CM coding in an ambulatory care encounter/visit either in a hospital clinic, outpatient surgical area, emergency room, physician's office, or other ambulatory care setting.
2. Sequence the ICD-9-CM code so that the first diagnosis shown in the medical record is the one chiefly responsible for the outpatient services provided during the encounter/visit.
3. Code the secondary diagnoses as follows:
   A. Chronic diseases that are treated on an ongoing basis may be coded and reported as many times as the patient receives treatment and care for the condition(s).
   B. Code all documented conditions that coexist at the time of the encounter/visit that require or affect patient care, treatment, or management.
   C. Conditions previously treated and no longer existing should not be coded.
4. Do not assign External Cause of Injury and Poisoning Codes (E codes), except those that identify the causative substance for an adverse effect of a drug that is correctly prescribed and properly administered (E930–E949).
5. Do not assign Morphology codes (M codes).
6. Do not assign ICD-9-CM procedure codes.
7. Assign CPT codes for all surgical procedures that fall in the surgery section.

8. Assign CPT codes from the following *only if* indicated on the case cover sheet:
   A. Anesthesia section
   B. Medicine section
   C. Evaluation and Management Services section
   D. Radiology section
   E. Laboratory and Pathology section
9. Assign CPT/HCPCS modifiers for hospital-based facilities, if applicable (regardless of payer).
10. Do not assign HCPCS Level II (alphanumeric) codes.

Inpatient Coding

1. Apply UDDS definitions, ICD-9-CM instructional notations and conventions, and current approved national ICD-9-CM coding guidelines to assign correct ICD-9-CM diagnostic and procedural codes to hospital inpatient medical records.
2. Sequence the ICD-9-CM codes, listing the principal diagnosis first.
3. Code other diagnoses that coexist at the time of admission, that develop subsequently, or that affect the treatment received and/or the length of stay. These represent additional conditions that affect patient care in terms of requiring clinical evaluation, therapeutic treatment, diagnostic procedures, extended length of hospital stay, or increased nursing care and/or monitoring.
   A. Code diagnoses that require active intervention during hospitalization. For example: Admission for small-bowel ileus and subsequent aspiration pneumonia that is treated with antibiotics and respiratory therapy. Code the ileus and aspiration pneumonia.
   B. Code diagnoses that require active management of chronic disease during hospitalization, which is defined as a patient who continues on chronic management at time of hospitalization. For example: Admission for acute exacerbation of COPD. The patient has depression that extends the stay and for which psychiatric consultation is obtained. Code the COPD and depression. For example: Admission for acute exacerbation of COPD. Physician lists "history of depression" on the Face Sheet, and the patient is given Desyrel. Code the COPD and depression.
   C. Code diagnoses of chronic systemic or generalized conditions that are not under active management when a physician documents them in the record and that may have a bearing on the management of the patient. For example: Admission for breast mass; diagnosis is carcinoma. Patient is blind and requires increased care. Code the breast carcinoma and blindness.
   D. Code status post previous surgeries or conditions likely to recur that may have a bearing on the management of the patient. For example: Admission for pneumonia; status post cardiac bypass surgery. Code the pneumonia and status post cardiac bypass surgery (V code).

E. Do not code status post previous surgeries or histories of conditions that have no bearing on the management of the patient. For example: Admission for pneumonia; status post hernia repair six months prior to admission. Code only the pneumonia.

F. Do not code localized conditions that have no bearing on the management of the patient. For example: Admission for hernia repair; the patient has a nevus on his leg that is not treated or evaluated. Code only the hernia and its repair.

G. Do not code abnormal findings (laboratory, x-ray, pathologic, and other diagnostic results) unless there is documentary evidence from the physician of their clinical significance. For example: Admission for elective joint replacement for degenerative joint disease. The laboratory report shows a serum sodium of 133; no further documentation addresses this laboratory result. Code only the degenerative joint disease and the replacement surgery. For example: Admission for elective joint replacement for degenerative joint disease. The laboratory report shows a low potassium level, and the physician documents hypokalemia. Intravenous potassium was administered by the physician for hypokalemia. Code the degenerative joint disease, the replacement surgery, and hypokalemia.

H. Do not code symptoms and signs that are characteristic of a diagnosis. For example: A patient has dyspnea due to COPD. Code only the COPD.

I. Do not code condition(s) in the Social History section that has no bearing on the management of the patient.

4. Do not assign External Cause of Injury and Poisoning Codes (E codes), except those that identify the causative substance for an adverse effect of a drug that is correctly prescribed and properly administered (E930–E949).

5. Do not assign Morphology codes (M codes).

6. Code all procedures that fall within the code range 01.01 through 86.99, but do not code 57.94 (Foley catheter).

7. Do not code procedures that fall within the code range 87.01 through 99.99. But code procedures in the following ranges:

87.51–87.54	Cholangiograms
87.74 and 87.76	Retrogrades, urinary systems
88.40–88.58	Arteriography and angiography
92.21–92.29	Radiation therapy
94.24–94.27	Psychiatric therapy
94.61–94.69	Alcohol/drug detoxification and rehabilitation
96.04	Insertion of endotracheal tube
96.70–96.72	Mechanical ventilation
98.51–98.59	ESWL
99.25	Hemotherapy

ICD-9-CM Coding Practice

Answers can be found in the back of this book in the Coding Practice Answer Key.

Infectious and Parasitic Diseases

1. Human immunodeficiency virus (HIV) with staphylococcal pneumonia
2. Admission for inguinal hernia repair. This 30-year-old patient has acquired immunodeficiency syndrome (AIDS) but is not symptomatic due to medication regimen. The procedure performed was a right indirect inguinal herniorrhaphy.
3. *Eschericia coli,* urosepsis

Endocrine, Nutritional, and Metabolic Diseases and Immunity Disorders

1. Diabetic ulcer of the right heel
2. Hypothyroidism due to thyroidectomy 7 years ago. Synthroid was given during hospitalization.
3. A 75-year-old male patient was admitted from a nursing home with dehydration and dysphagia due to a previous stroke. During hospitalization the patient was rehydrated and transferred back to the nursing home.

Mental Disorder

1. Bipolar disorder
2. Major depression, single episode, severe with psychosis
3. A patient is admitted to an acute care facility for detoxification from alcohol intoxication and barbiturate abuse with chronic alcoholism and barbiturate abuse. The patient also has cirrhosis of the liver due to alcoholism.

Diseases of the Blood and Blood Forming Organs, Nervous System and Sense Organs

1. A 45-year-old woman is admitted for blood loss anemia due to a chronic, hemorrhagic, recurrent gastric ulcer. The patient is given a blood transfusion and her oral Tagamet is continued.
2. Repetitive seizures with tic douloreux
3. Mature senile cataract; diabetes mellitus with hypertension and acute renal failure
4. An 84-year-old woman was admitted with hemiplegia and aphasia. A CT scan of the brain was performed which revealed an acute cerebral infarction. The patient was discharged with a final diagnosis of acute cerebral infarction.

Diseases of the Respiratory System

1. A patient was admitted with a temperature of 102 and atrial fibrillation. The chest x-ray reveals pneumonia with subsequent documentation by the physician of pneumonia in the progress notes and discharge summary. The patient was treated with oral antiarrhythmia medications and IV antibiotics.
2. Acute exacerbation of COPD with stage V hypertensive kidney disease.
3. A patient is admitted with respiratory failure, hypertension, and congestive heart failure.

Diseases of the Digestive System

1. Esophageal varices with cirrhosis and hemorrhage
2. A patient is admitted to the hospital complaining of abdominal pain. Following evaluation it was determined that the patient had an intestinal obstruction due to adhesions from a prior abdominal surgery. The patient underwent an exploratory laparotomy with lysis of adhesions.
3. A patient with chronic cholecystitis and gallbladder stones underwent a laparoscopic cholecystectomy. However, due to extensive gallbladder adhesions the procedure was converted to an open cholecystectomy.
4. A patient with a family history of colon cancer was admitted for a screening colonoscopy. During the colonoscopy, polyps of the colon were found and a polypectomy performed.

Diseases of the Genitourinary System

1. A patient is admitted with hydronephrosis and a staghorn calculus of the kidney. The patient underwent a ureteroscopy with placement of ureteral stents and removal of calculus.
2. A female patient is admitted for a second-degree cystocele. An anterior repair is performed.

Diseases of Skin and Subcutaneous Tissue

1. A 77-year-old nursing home patient was admitted for excisional debridement of decubitus ulcer via surgical excision in the OR of the heel. The patient also has degenerative joint disease of both knees.
2. Venomous snake bite of the ankle, three days prior to encounter, with cellulitis
3. Cyst of skin of right arm with excision
4. Malignant melanoma of the back, wide excision of the melanoma

Diseases of the Musculoskeletal System and Connective Tissue

1. Displacement of lumbar intervertebral disk treated with a laminectomy and diskectomy
2. Compression fracture of the sacral vertebrae due to osteoporosis

Complications of Pregnancy and Childbirth Complications, Abortion, Congenital Anomalies, and Perinatal Conditions

1. Normal pregnancy and delivery with loose nuchal cord around neck and episiotomy with delivery of liveborn male infant. Delivery room record states "no evidence of fetal problem."
2. Term live birth delivery with macrosomia and hemorrhage following episiotomy with low forceps delivery prior to expulsion of the placenta.
3. Twin delivery at 32 weeks. Both babies were delivered vaginally and were liveborn.
4. Cephalic presentation with vaginal delivery resulting in a single liveborn female. Episiotomy with episiorrhaphy.
5. Fallopian tube pregnancy with salpingectomy
6. A patient admitted with vaginal bleeding and a miscarriage is treated with aspiration dilation and curettage of uterus.
7. A patient is readmitted for renal failure following completed treatment for a miscarriage three weeks ago.
8. Atrial septal defect
9. Term male infant with facial laceration due to scalpel from Cesarean section
10. Single, liveborn, term male infant delivered in the hospital at 36 weeks
11. Twin newborns, both born premature at 32 weeks via Cesarean section, 1,002 g was the weight of the first twin whose mate was stillborn. The baby was admitted to the nursery from the delivery room. The baby also was treated for jaundice due to ABO incompatibility.

Disease of the Circulatory System

1. A patient is admitted to the acute care facility with chest pain. The patient was awakened from sleep; this was the patient's first experience with chest pain. The patient was given two nitroglycerin tablets in the emergency department. The chest pain was not relieved, resulting in the diagnosis of angina. Serial CPK was normal. Following a cardiac catheterization, the patient is found to have arteriosclerotic coronary artery disease.
2. Acute pulmonary edema with congestive heart failure
3. Congestive heart failure with hypertension
4. A 64-year-old female was discharged with the final diagnosis of acute renal failure and hypertension.

Neoplasms

1. This is the first admission for a patient with adenocarcinoma of the right lower lung with metastasis to the brain. The patient underwent a lobectomy.
2. The patient was admitted for breast carcinoma in the right breast at two o'clock. This was removed via lumpectomy. The patient was found to have 1 of 7 lymph nodes positive for carcinoma during axillary lymph node dissection.
3. Stage III carcinoma of the prostate with metastatic disease to the liver. The patient underwent a bilateral orchiectomy.
4. A terminal ovarian cancer patient is admitted with severe dehydration. She was diagnosed with ovarian cancer three years ago and has peritoneal carcinomatosis with malignant ascites. She was rehydrated and discharged.
5. A patient is admitted with a chronic productive cough with hemoptysis. A transbronchial bronchoscopy with biopsy of the lower lobe was undertaken that revealed squamous cell carcinoma.
6. Carcinoma of the multiple overlapping sites of the bladder. The patient underwent transurethral fulguration of bladder lesions.
7. A patient has metastatic adenocarcinoma of bone.
8. A patient has squamous cell carcinoma of the knee.
9. A patient is admitted with metastatic carcinoma from breast to liver with previous mastectomy with no reoccurrence at the primary site.
10. Metastatic carcinoma of the lung

Injuries

1. A policeman on duty was hit in the eye with a bat. In the emergency department, the patient was diagnosed with a hyphema.
2. Right orbital roof fracture
3. A patient was admitted after a fall down a series of steps. The patient was unconscious for approximately 45 minutes. A skull vault fracture with cerebral contusion was found on CT scan.
4. Torn lateral meniscus of the right knee
5. A young woman was admitted after a car hit her from behind while she waited for a bus. She sustained a fractured fibula shaft and patella with a break in the skin at the mid-calf. The patient required an open reduction of the fibula fracture.

Burns

1. Second- and first-degree burns of the upper thigh
2. Second- and third-degree burns of the abdomen with 25 percent of the body burned with 15 percent of the body having third-degree burns

Poisoning and Adverse Effects of Drugs

1. Syncope; bradycardia ruled out; due to taking Valium as prescribed by a physician. The patient also took an antihistamine as directed on the package, without consulting a healthcare provider.
2. A patient was given heparin during hospitalization for a deep vein thrombophlebitis of the right lower extremity. The patient had back pain and the nurse was not answering the bell, so he decided to take two aspirin. The interaction between the aspirin and the heparin caused a subcutaneous hemorrhage of the thigh of the lower right extremity.
3. Suicide attempt with overdose of Percocet
4. Drug reaction to an antihistamine taken and prescribed correctly

Complications of Surgical and Medical Care

1. Displacement of prosthetic femoral head
2. Pain due to pacemaker electrode
3. Intraoperative cerebral infarction
4. Postoperative pulmonary edema
5. Sepsis due to the presence of an indwelling urinary catheter with a positive culture reflected in the progress notes of *Staphylococcus aureus* sepsis
6. Postoperative transplant rejection following heart transplant

CPT Coding Practice

Answers can be found in the back of this book in the Coding Practice Answer Key.

Anesthesia

Please code the appropriate *anesthesia* code for the following procedures:

1. Removal of cataract, ASA of 2
2. Tracheotomy in 3-month-old patient
3. Radical mastectomy
4. Insertion central venous pressure (CVP) for venous access catheter 00532
5. Lumbar sympathectomy
6. EGD
7. Menisectomy of the knee, ASA 3
8. Open reduction fracture of the distal ulna
9. Cardiac catheterization
10. Vaginal delivery

Medicine

1. Tetanus immune globulin IM
2. Vaccination for hepatitis A and hepatitis B, adult, IM
3. Chemotherapy for 3 hours' infusion
4. Esophageal acid reflux test
5. Right and left cardiac catheterization retrograde approach with angiography and ventriculography

Radiology

1. Chest x-ray, two views
2. Chest x-ray, complete
3. Abdominal ultrasound, complete
4. Mammogram of right breast
5. Screening mammogram
6. Mammographic guidance for breast needle localization placement
7. CT scan guidance for liver biopsy
8. Ultrasound of kidneys, complete
9. CT scan of head with contrast
10. MRI of chest without contrast

Surgery—Integumentary

1. Wide excision of 0.65-cm melanoma (margins included) from right forearm
2. Excision of two (2) left breast lesions
3. Excision of basal cell carcinoma, 1.9-cm lesion left upper eyelid
4. Removal of two (2) skin tags on chest (0.3 cm and 0.5 cm)
5. Repair of laceration of left thigh (5.1 cm) with suture of epidermis and dermis
6. Repair of two (2) wounds of the neck (2.0 cm and 1.4 cm) with layered closure

Surgery—Musculoskeletal

1. Surgical arthroscopy of the left shoulder with decompression and acromioplasty
2. Closed reduction of fracture of right proximal ulna
3. Hallux valgus repair with resection of the joint with implant in the first left toe proximal phalanx
4. Open reduction with internal fixation of right humeral condylar lateral fracture
5. Diagnostic arthroscopy of left knee with medial and lateral meniscus repair
6. Removal of pins and screws from right ankle following open reduction and internal fixation occurring 1 year ago
7. Posterior fasciotomy for compartment syndrome of left upper leg following recent trauma

Surgery—Respiratory

1. Extensive excision of bilateral nasal polyps
2. Endoscopic sinusotomy with bilateral anterior ethmoidectomy
3. Bronchoscopy with bilateral transbronchial biopsy
4. Thoracoscopic pleurodesis
5. Indirect laryngoscopic removal of foreign body
6. Thoracoscopic left thoracic sympathectomy
7. Percutaneous biopsy of the right lung

Surgery—Cardiovascular/Lymph

1. Percutaneous balloon angioplasty of renal artery
2. Diagnostic left and right retrograde heart catheterization through left heart cath, left ventriculogram, coronary arteriogram
3. Replacement of dual chamber pacemaker generator with removal of old generator
4. Creation of arteriovenous anastomosis for renal dialysis, open; by basilic vein transposition

Surgery—Digestive

1. Rubber band hemorrhoidectomy of external hemorrhoids
2. Esophagogastroduodenoscopy with sclerotherapy of esophageal varices
3. Esophagogastroduodenoscopy with insertion of percutaneous endoscopic gastrostomy
4. Colonoscopy with cauterization of diverticular bleeding
5. Sigmoidoscopy with snare removal of polyp
6. Laparoscopic recurrent left inguinal hernia repair
7. A 3-year-old male undergoes repair of an initial incarcerated right inguinal hernia

Surgery—Genitourinary

1. Cystourethroscopy with removal of 1.5-cm bladder tumor
2. Cystourethroscopy with removal of ureteral calculus
3. Cystoscopy with insertion of double-J ureteral stent in right ureter
4. Transurethral resection of the prostate with electrocautery
5. Laparoscopic sling procedure for urinary incontinence
6. Circumcision of 32-year-old male using clamp
7. Cryosurgical destruction of simple papilloma of the penis
8. Endoscopic laser destruction of endometriosis of ovary and cul-de-sac
9. Laparoscopic tubal ligation
10. Ovarian cystectomy
11. Hysteroscopy with endometrial ablation
12. Laparoscopic salpingectomy for removal of ectopic pregnancy
13. Dilatation and curettage for missed abortion at 11 weeks' gestation
14. Removal of cervical cerclage under spinal anesthesia in a pregnant woman

Surgery—Nervous

1. Blood patch for postspinal headache
2. Bilateral epidural lumbar injection of steroids

Surgery—Ocular/Auditory

1. Repair of oval window fistula
2. Extraction of extracapsular cataract with simultaneous intraocular lens insertion in the right eye
3. Endolaser photocoagulation repair of retinal detachment in the left eye

Evaluation and Management Mapping Practice

The following map shows how a given facility has determined the criteria for evaluation and management (E/M) code assignment based on an emergency department record. Use the map to determine the correct codes for the emergency record that is provided. *Remember that each facility has the ability to develop its own mapping strategy. Therefore, the mapping scenario for the CCS Examination will most likely be different from this one.* The purpose of this exercise is to practice using any mapping criteria that you are provided during the national examination.

Points Needed to Determine the Level of CPT Code

Level 1 = 1–20
Level 2 = 21–35
Level 3 = 36–47
Level 4 = 48–60
Level 5 = $\geq$ 61
Critical Care $\geq$ 61 with constant physician attendance

CPT Codes

Level 1	99281	99281–25 with procedure/laboratory/radiology
Level 2	99282	99282–25 with procedure/laboratory/radiology
Level 3	99283	99283–25 with procedure/laboratory/radiology
Level 4	99284	99284–25 with procedure/laboratory/radiology
Level 5	99285	99285–25 with procedure/laboratory/radiology

Emergency Department Acuity Points

	5	10	15	20	25
Meds Given	0–2	3–5	6–7	8–9	> 10
Extent of Hx	Brief	PF	EPF	Detail	Comprehensive
Extent of Examination	Brief	PF	EPF	Detail	Comprehensive
# of Tests Ordered	0–1	2–3	4–5	6–7	> 8
Supplies Used	1	2–3	4–5	6–7	> 8

SAMPLE EMERGENCY DEPARTMENT RECORD

DATE OF ADMISSION: 6/19 **DATE OF DISCHARGE:** 6/19

HISTORY (Problem Focused):

ADMISSION HISTORY: This 45-year-old African-American male was working in his office when he received news that his daughter, who is in the military, was deployed emergently to the Middle East. He began to have sharp pain in his right chest.

ALLERGIES: None

CHRONIC MEDICATIONS: None

FAMILY HISTORY: Noncontributory

SOCIAL HISTORY: The patient smokes one pack of cigarettes per day but he does not smoke in the house.

REVIEW OF SYSTEMS: His integumentary, musculoskeletal, cardiovascular, genitourinary, and gastrointestinal systems are negative.

PHYSICAL EXAMINATION (Extended Problem Focused):

GENERAL APPEARANCE: This is an alert cooperative male in acute distress.

HEENT: PERRLA, extraocular movements are full

NECK: Supple

CHEST: Lungs are clear without rales or rhonchi. Heart has normal sinus rhythm.

ABDOMEN: Soft and nontender, no organomegaly

EXTREMITIES: Examination is normal

LABORATORY DATA: Urinalysis is normal, EKG normal, chest x-ray is normal. CBC and diff, cardiac enzymes show no abnormalities.

IMPRESSION: Noncardiac chest pain

TREATMENT: The patient was reassured, counseled to stop smoking, and referred to the clinic for smoking cessation and further management.

DISCHARGE DIAGNOSES: Noncardiac chest pain, possible anxiety reaction, smoking.

DISCHARGE INSTRUCTIONS: The patient was instructed to make an appointment for the clinic tomorrow.

Questions

1. What is the diagnostic code?
2. What CPT code would you use based on the mapping scenario?

(For answers, see the Answer Key for Coding Practice.)

Test Taking

The multiple choice section of the CCS exam is important because those who take the exam must pass both the multiple choice section as well as the cases. If either section is failed, the candidate will not pass the national examination. Because of this scoring methodology, candidates must study well for the multiple choice section. Practice by answering the multiple choice questions and evaluate any areas with which you do not have familiarity. List or highlight the areas that are unfamiliar to you and strategize how you will research these areas.

MS-DRGs

Obtain the MS-DRG list for fiscal year 2008 (refer to the Study Resources section in the Introduction). Highlight the most common MS-DRGs that will occur in the average hospital and look at how they are ordered. This type of study will help you in several ways. You become familiar with the most common MS-DRGs and see the hierarchy of MS-DRG decision trees. Generally, the MS-DRG grouper considers the following information: whether the patient had a procedure, the age of the patient, and whether there was a major comorbid condition (MCC). The answer of "yes" or "no" to these questions determines the MS-DRG. There are Web sites and books from AHIMA that will further explain MS-DRG decision trees and other issues such as case mix analysis. See the resource section of this book for more information.

It is important to review the definitions of case mix and case mix analysis.

- **Case mix**: Total of all the DRG weights of the patients seen in a given facility over a particular time period.
- **Case mix index**: Average weight of all cases seen (total weights divided by the number of patients).

Ambulatory Payment Classifications (APCs)

It is important to understand the methodology of APCs. Some important issues to review are discounting, impact of CPT and HCPCS codes, medical necessity, the Correct Coding Initiative (CCI), status indicators, packaging, and the three-year transitional corridor. Refer to the "Coding Challenges: Review and Guides" chapter in this book. AHIMA also has excellent resources regarding this topic. You should also visit the CMS Web site for Medicare Program Memorandum.

Health Insurance Portability and Accountability Act (HIPAA)

Review recent AHIMA practice briefs and articles on this topic. Questions about HIPAA could be present in the multiple choice section of the examination. An easy way to study this area is to access information from the Body of Knowledge in the AHIMA CoP.

Sample Multiple Choice Questions

Part I of the CCS examination consists of 60 four-option, multiple choice questions. You will have one hour to complete the multiple choice section during the examination. Please note that you are not permitted to use your code books for this section of the examination.

Please circle the best answer for the following questions. Answers are in the Answers for Practice Coding.

1. Hospital A: The patient is admitted for chest pain and is found to have an acute inferior myocardial infarction with atrial fibrillation. After the atrial fibrillation was controlled and the patient was stabilized, the patient was transferred to Hospital B for a CABG X3. The appropriate sequencing and ICD codes for both hospitalizations would be:

   410.41 Myocardial infarction of inferior wall, initial episode
   410.42 Myocardial infarction of inferior wall, subsequent episode
   410.91 Myocardial infarction, initial episode
   410.92 Myocardial infarction, subsequent episode
   427.31 Atrial fibrillation
   786.50 Chest pain
   36.13 Aortocoronary bypass of three coronary arteries

   A. Hospital A: 786.50, 410.91, 427.31; Hospital B; 410.92, 36.13
   B. Hospital A: 410.41, 427.31; Hospital B; 410.92, 36.13
   C. Hospital A: 410.41, 427.31; Hospital B; 410.41, 36.13
   D. Hospital A: 410.42, 427.31; Hospital B; 410.41, 36.13

2. The patient was admitted from the emergency department because of chest pain. Following blood work it was determined that the CPK was elevated with MB enzymes elevated. The EKG shows nonspecific ST changes. What type of diagnosis may this be indicative of?

   A. Unstable angina
   B. Myocardial infarction
   C. Congestive heart failure
   D. Mitral valve stenosis

3. A patient is seen in the emergency department for chest pain. After evaluation of the patient it is suspected that the patient may have gastroesophageal reflux disease (GERD). The final diagnosis was "rule out chest pain versus GERD." The correct code is:

   A. Admission for suspected cardiovascular condition (V71.7)
   B. Esophageal pain (789.01)
   C. Gastrointestinal reflux (530.81)
   D. Chest pain NOS (786.50)

Please refer to the following when answering questions 4 and 5.

216.0	Benign Neoplasm of Skin	
	Includes:	Blue Nevus
		Dermatofibroma
		Hydrocystoma
		Pigmented Nevus
		Syringoadenoma
		Syringoma
	Excludes:	
		Skin of genital organs (221.–222.9)

4. When coding benign neoplasm of the skin, the section noted above directs the coder to:
   A. Use category 216 for a syringoma
   B. Use category 216 for malignant melanoma
   C. Use category 216 for malignant neoplasm of the bone
   D. Use category 216 for malignant neoplasm of the skin

5. When coding benign neoplasm of the skin of the labia, the section noted above directs the coder to:
   A. Use category 216
   B. Use category 221.0–222.9
   C. Use category 174
   D. Use category 173

6. If a patient has a principal diagnosis of septicemia, which of the following procedures will increase the DRG assignment the most?
   A. Bronchoscopy with biopsy
   B. Excisional débridement of nails
   C. Excisional débridement of skin ulcer with abrasion
   D. Ventilator management for less than 96 hours

7. A patient presents to a facility with a history of prostate cancer, and with mental confusion on admission. The patient completed radiation therapy for prostatic carcinoma three years ago and is status post a radical resection of the prostate. A CT scan of the brain reveals metastatic carcinoma of the brain. The correct coding and sequencing of this patient's record is:
   A. Metastatic carcinoma of the brain; carcinoma of the prostate; mental confusion
   B. Mental confusion; history of carcinoma of the prostate; admission for chemotherapy
   C. Metastatic carcinoma of the brain; history of carcinoma of the prostate
   D. Carcinoma of the prostate; metastatic carcinoma to the brain

8. Carcinoma of multiple overlapping sites of the bladder. Diagnostic cystoscopy and transurethral fulguration of bladder lesions (1.9 cm, 6.0 cm) are undertaken. The appropriate CPT code(s) would be:

   52000 Cystourethroscopy

   52224 Cystourethroscopy, with fulguration (including cryosurgery or treatment of) minor (less than 0.5 cm) tumor(s) with or without biopsy

   52234 Cystourethroscopy, with fulguration (including cryosurgery or treatment of) small (less than 0.5 cm to 2.0 cm) tumor(s) with or without biopsy

   52235 Cystourethroscopy, with fulguration (including cryosurgery or treatment of) medium (2.0 cm to 5.0 cm) tumor(s) with or without biopsy

   52240 Cystourethroscopy, with fulguration (including cryosurgery or treatment of) large bladder tumor(s) with or without biopsy

   A. 52234 and 52240

   B. 52235

   C. 52240

   D. 52000, 52234, 52260

9. The patient is discharged with hemiplegia and aphasia associated with a cerebral infarction of the left side of the brain. The patient is right handed. The patient also has compensated congestive heart failure and a history of hypertension (both conditions currently controlled on medication and treated while in the hospital). What code assignment would be appropriate?

   342.90 Hemiparesis affecting unspecified side

   342.91 Hemiparesis affecting dominant side

   342.92 Hemiparesis affecting nondominant side

   434.90 Cerebral artery occlusion unspecified

   434.91 Cerebral artery occlusion with infarction

   401.9 Hypertension

   428.0 Congestive heart failure

   784.3 Aphasia

   A. 434.91, 342.91, 784.3, 428.0, 401.9

   B. 342.90, 784.3, 428.0, 401.9

   C. 434.90, 342.90, 784.3

   D. 434.91, 342.90, 784.3

10. A laparoscopic tubal ligation is undertaken. What is the correct CPT code assignment?

49320	Laparoscopy, surgical; with biopsy (single or multiple)
58662	Laparoscopy, surgical; with fulguration or excision of lesions of the ovary, pelvic viscera, or peritoneal surface by any method
58670	Laparoscopy, surgical; with fulguration of oviducts (with or without transection)
58671	Laparoscopy, surgical; with occlusion of oviducts (with or without transection)

A. 49320, 58662

B. 58670

C. 58671

D. 49320

11. A patient's principal diagnosis is pneumonia (486). Which of the following may legitimately change the coding of the pneumonia in accordance with the UHDDS and relevant clinical medicine if appropriately documented?

A. Sputum culture reflects growth of normal flora

B. Patient has a positive Gram stain

C. Patient is found to have dysphagia with aspiration

D. Patient has nonproductive sputum

12. A patient was admitted for abdominal pain with diarrhea and was diagnosed with infectious gastroenteritis. The patient also had angina and chronic obstructive pulmonary disease. The diagnoses would be coded and sequenced as:

A. Abdominal pain; infectious gastroenteritis; chronic obstructive pulmonary disease; angina

B. Infectious gastroenteritis; chronic obstructive pulmonary disease; angina

C. Gastroenteritis; abdominal pain; angina

D. Diarrhea; chronic obstructive pulmonary disease; angina

Sample Cases

SAMPLE INPATIENT CASE

DATE OF ADMISSION: 1/5 **DATE OF DISCHARGE:** 1/7

DISCHARGE DIAGNOSIS:

1. Adenocarcinoma of the endometrium
2. Hemoperitoneum
3. Postoperative hemorrhage
4. Hemorrhagic shock secondary to blood loss

COURSE IN HOSPITAL: The patient was taken to the operating room on 1/5 where a laparoscopically assisted vaginal hysterectomy was carried out.

At approximately 6:30 p.m. on the same day, I was called back into the hospital's recovery room because the patient was in shock with blood pressure of 80/60 with poor urine output and distended abdomen.

At this point it was decided to do an emergency diagnostic laparoscopy with preoperative diagnosis of postoperative hemorrhage. Bleeders were controlled with hemostatic sutures applied through the laparoscope.

The immediate postoperative course was essentially stormy with urine output maintained at 30 mL/h.

An ultrasound of the abdomen and pelvis was requested on the second postoperative day and this revealed normal renal shadow; no abnormal fluid accumulation in the pelvis or in the abdominal wall. The patient was then transferred to the regular floor on 1/6 after having maintained a satisfactory postoperative course from the second surgical procedure. The Jackson-Pratt drain was removed on 1/7 with closure of the abdominal incision with Steri-strips. The patient remained afebrile. She had been out of bed with good urine output and tolerating house diet. Her activities were increased gradually. Hemoglobin was again checked prior to discharge and was 12.1 g.

The patient was discharged to home on 1/7.

INSTRUCTIONS ON DISCHARGE: Regular diet. Follow up with appointment in my office in 3 days and with a colonoscopy for colon screening in light of family history of colon cancer.

HISTORY AND PHYSICAL EXAMINATION

ADMITTED: 1/5

REASON FOR ADMISSION: Vaginal bleeding

HISTORY OF PRESENT ILLNESS: This is a 62-year-old white female, gravida IV, para IV. She states that she has been in good health and has not had any gynecological complaints. During the past year she has had some left lower-quadrant pain and has noted post-coital bleeding. The bleeding has also occurred on and off for several months.

PAST MEDICAL HISTORY: Hypothyroidism due to thyroidectomy many years ago for benign tumor. No other serious illnesses, operations, or hospitalizations. The patient takes Synthroid .200 mcg.

ALLERGIES: No known drug or food allergies.

CHRONIC MEDICATIONS: Synthroid .200 mcg

FAMILY HISTORY: Her mother died of colon cancer at age 53 years.

SOCIAL HISTORY: The patient is married with four children. She does not drink or smoke.

REVIEW OF SYSTEMS: HEENT essentially negative; wears glasses. Cardiorespiratory; no cough, dyspnea, cyanosis or chest pain. Gastrointestinal; no specific digestive or bowel complaints, with the exception of the non-specific left lower quadrant pain. The patient has no specific urinary complaints. The patient has a low hemoglobin level.

PHYSICAL EXAMINATION:

GENERAL APPEARANCE: Well-developed, well-nourished 62-year-old woman in no acute distress

HEENT: Essentially negative

LUNGS: Clear to P & A

HEART: Regular in force, rate, and rhythm. There are no audible murmurs.

ABDOMEN: No hernia or palpable masses. Abdomen is soft and flat. Peristalsis is normal. There are no areas of tenderness.

GENITALIA: Bimanual examination reveals the external genitalia to be normal. The uterus is of normal size. There are no palpable pelvic masses or tenderness.

RECTAL: Negative

IMPRESSION: Postmenopausal bleeding, possible endometrial carcinoma with blood loss anemia

PLAN: Vaginal hysterectomy

PROGRESS NOTES

DATE	NOTE
1/5	The patient is admitted for LAVH because of postmenopausal bleeding. She has also had left lower-quadrant pain. General condition is good. Operative Note: Preop: Possible adenocarcinoma of the endometrium Postop: Same, pathology pending Procedure: LAVH Anesthesia: General

Findings: Tubes and ovaries were within normal limits. Uterus is submitted for pathologic examination.

EBL 300 ccs

Called back to the RR for decrease in blood pressure and decreased urine output. The patient was found to have abdominal distention as well. The patient was given 3 units of blood and taken back to the operating room for evaluation of postoperative hemorrhage.

Operative note:

Preop: Postop hemorrhage

Postop: Accidental laceration of epigastric artery, acute blood loss anemia

Procedure: Repair of bleeding vessel via laparoscope

Anesthesia: General

EBL: 1,500 to 2,000 mL of blood

The patient was admitted to the ICU following surgery where we will monitor her progress throughout the night.

1/6 Patient is doing well today. The BP is stable, urine output good—diuresing well, wound clean and dry, healing well. Will transfer her to the surgical floor.

1/7 The patient is stable, offers no complaints. Will discharge to home.

PHYSICIAN'S ORDERS

DATE	ORDER
1/5	Admit for LAVH
	Type and cross 4 units of blood, CBC
	Prepare for vaginal hysterectomy
	Synthroid .200 mcg daily
	NPO
	Demerol 75 mg
	Atropin 0.4 mg preop
	Postop, transfer patient to ICU
	D5NSS 125 cc/h
	Transfuse three units PRBC
	Demerol 75 mg IM q. 4 hours as need for pain.
	Ancef 500 mg q. 6 hrs × 3 doses
	CBC q. 4 hrs, Strict I & O
1/6	Transfer to floor, Please get patient OOB and provide liquids at bedside
	Continue I & O
	CBC this a.m. then tomorrow a.m.
	D/C IV after 6:00 p.m. if stable
1/7	Discharge to home

OPERATIVE REPORT

DATE: 1/5

PREOPERATIVE DIAGNOSIS: Possible adenocarcinoma of the endometrium

POSTOPERATIVE DIAGNOSIS: Pending pathology report

OPERATION: Laparoscopic assisted vaginal hysterectomy with pelvic cytology

ANESTHESIA: General

OPERATIVE PROCEDURE: With the patient under satisfactory general anesthesia in the semilithotomy position, she was prepped and draped in the usual fashion for a laparoscopic and vaginal procedure. Through an infraumbilical incision, a Veress needle was inserted to establish a pneumoperitoneum using a high-flow insufflator with CO_2 gas, maintaining 15 mm of pressure. It was then followed by insertion of a 10-mm trocar into the infraumbilical incision, followed by the laparoscope with laparoscopic examination having been done with findings described above.

After transillumination of the abdomen noting vessels, an incision was made in the skin and 12-mm trocars and sleeves were inserted into the right and left lower quadrant.

After having inserted the 12-mm sleeves, an endogauge was inserted into Channel A and levels of the right and left tubo-ovarian ligaments and broad ligaments were measured. An endo-GIA was then inserted into Channel A, followed by endo-GIA of Channel B, amputating the attachments of the tubes and ovaries and the broad ligaments. The remaining attachments of the board ligaments and the round ligaments were picked up with endo-GIA staplers on both sides.

A grasper was then inserted on Channel A, and the bladder reflection was picked up and elevated. It was then opened with endoshears, and using hydrodissection and ultrasonic scalpel, a bladder flap was created by sharp and blunt dissection with the scalpel. The dissection was carried down to the surface of the anterior lip of the cervix, which was noted to be smooth and free of adhesions. This was extended down past the cervicovaginal junction with identification of the tenaculum in the vagina. The grasper was then replaced on the right cornua and traction placed on the uterus, exposing the right cardinal ligaments, which was then placed on traction and using the scalpel probe, skeletonization of the uterine arteries with exposure of the arteries was done automatically.

The peritoneum was then dissected down past the uterosacral ligament insertion. After complete skeletonization of the uterine arteries was done, an endo TA-30 stapler was placed on the uterine arteries and the pedicle was cut off with the scalpel. There were no bleeding points noted.

OPERATIVE REPORT

The grasper was then removed and inserted into Channel B, and the left cornua of the uterus was picked up and placed on traction. The left cardinal ligaments and uterine arteries were then picked up and skeletonized, and complete exposure and dissection was done with visualization and identification of the arteries. The fragments of paravesical tissue were dissected off with the scalpel without traumatizing the bladder, which had previously been filled up with methylene blue and no spillage of the dye was noted during dissection of the uterus.

An endo TA-30 was then inserted in Channel A and linear staples were placed on the uterine arteries, on the left uterine artery and the cardinal ligament pedicles. The pedicle was then cut off with the scalpel. A second line of staples was then placed below the first line, taking care not to include the dome of the bladder without entering the vagina, and the pedicle cut off with the scalpel. There was a change in color of the uterus from pink to gray, indicating complete obliteration of blood supply.

The staple lines on the infundibular pelvis ligaments were then inspected and this was found to be adequate. At this time the laparoscopic procedure was temporarily stopped and attention was then paid to the vaginal portion of the procedure, releasing the pneumoperitoneum that had been established for the laparoscopy. The cervix was exposed and picked up on the anterior a posterior lip with Lahey clamps, and a circumscribing incision was made on the cervicovaginal junction down to the level of the paravesical fascia and dissected off by sharp and blunt dissection with entry into the anterior cul-de-sac atraumatically, and the posterior cul-de-sac entered likewise.

The insertions of the base of the uterosacral ligaments and cardinal ligaments were then picked up with Heaney clamps, cut and suture ligated with #0 Vicryl, followed by a second line of Heaney clamps on the base of the remaining portion of the cardinal ligaments that was attached to the uterus, amputating and freeing up the uterus. The pedicles were tied off with #0 Vicryl materials and the uterus pulled and delivered out of the abdominal cavity through the vagina. Angle sutures were then placed on the vaginal cuff using #0 Vicryl material, and the intervening incision was closed with vertical mattress sutures using #0 Vicryl material.

After having closed the vagina and establishing adequate hemostasis, attention was once again placed on the laparoscopic portion. The pneumoperitoneum was once again established using high-flow insufflator and CO_2 gas at 10-mm pressure, and inspection and irrigation of the vascular pedicles and the vaginal cuff was done, which revealed them to be dry. The pelvis was irrigated with copious amounts of warm saline solution. The procedure was then terminated. The sleeve and gripper in Channel A was removed, and was found to be dry. The fascia was closed using an endo close needle with a #0 Vicryl suture in interrupted fashion using three stitches. The channel B 12-mm sheath and trocar were removed, which were dry.

OPERATIVE REPORT

At this time, termination of the procedure was done. The laparoscope was removed and the CO_2 released gradually. All instruments were removed and remaining stab wounds were closed in the fascia with #0 Vicryl sutures, and subcutaneously with #4-0 Monocryl. Sterile dressings were applied.

The patient was transferred to the recovery room in a reactive state with stable vital signs. Estimated blood loss was 300 mL of whole blood, no replacement given.

PATHOLOGY REPORT

DATE: 1/5

SPECIMEN: Uterus

CLINICAL DATA:

Preoperative diagnosis: Adenocarcinoma of endometrium

Postoperative diagnosis: Same

GROSS DESCRIPTION: The specimen is labeled "Uterus." Submitted uterus with cervix attached. The specimen has previously been partially opened. It measures 9 × 5 × 3 cm and weight 58 g. The body of the uterus appears to be symmetrical. On section, the endocervix and ectocervix appear essentially normal. The endocervical canal likewise appears normal. The endometrial cavity is involved by a polypoid tumor mass chiefly in the right cornual area and measuring 3 cm in greatest diameter. The tumor appears to superficially penetrate the myometrium. The specimen will be further sectioned following fixation.

A and B are sections of cervix; C, D, E, F, G, and H are full-thickness section of tumor; section I is a full-thickness section from grossly uninvolved tissue.

MICROSCOPIC DESCRIPTION:

DIAGNOSIS: Adenocarcinoma, intermediate grade, of endometrium. Chronic cervicitis

COMMENT: The tumor penetrates approximately 0.4 cm into a total myometrial thickness of 1.5 cm.

OPERATIVE REPORT

DATE: 1/5

PREOPERATIVE DIAGNOSIS: Postoperative hemorrhage

POSTOPERATIVE DIAGNOSIS: Bleeding from right epigastric artery

OPERATION: Emergency diagnostic laparoscopy with repair of epigastric artery and blood transfusion

ANESTHESIA: General

OPERATIVE INDICATIONS: Estimated blood loss 1,500 to 2,000 mL of whole blood

OPERATIVE PROCEDURE: There was liquid and clotted blood in the abdominal cavity, approximately 1,500 to 2,000 mL, with blood coming from the puncture in the right lower quadrant, apparently from an accidental laceration of the right epigastric artery. The pedicles were inspected in the pelvis, and these were found to be dry.

With the patient under satisfactory general anesthesia, after having been transfused three units of packed RBCs, she was taken to the operating room and an emergency laparoscopic examination was carried out by opening the previous stab wounds with irrigation of the abdominal and pelvic cavity, evacuating approximately 1,500 to 2,000 mL of liquid and clotted blood.

Exposure of the pedicles of the infundibulopelvic ligament on both sides and the uterine arteries and the vaginal vault revealed them to be dry. There was no bleeding anywhere else in the pelvic cavity.

A puncture was found in the epigastric artery. Using an endoclosed needle through which a #0 Vicryl ligature was attached, the artery was repaired, stopping the bleeding point. This was verified by inspection with the laparoscope. After this was accomplished, the fascia was once again closed with endoclosed needle and #0 Vicryl suture on the right lower quadrant. The left lower quadrant was left open, and a Jackson-Pratt drain was inserted into the incision and placed in the pelvis for drainage.

The patient was then removed from the Trendelenburg position after ascertaining that vital signs were stable. The CO_2 was released gradually. All instruments were removed, and subcuticular closure of the stab wounds was done using #4-0 Monocryl sutures.

At the termination of surgery the patient's vital signs were stable. She, however, remained hypotensive with tachycardia with good urine output and was transfused an additional three units and transferred to the intensive care unit for postoperative care.

LABORATORY REPORTS

HEMATOLOGY

Specimen	Results				Normal Values
	1/5	1/5	1/5	1/5	
WBC	5.0	5.0	5.2	5.1	4.3–11.0
RBC	5.0	4.0L	4.2L	4.5	4.5–5.9
HGB	7.1L	5.5L	7.9L	9.0L	13.5–17.5
HCT	38L	32L	39L	43	41–52
MCV	90	89	97	96	80–100
MCHC	44	46	48	50	31–57
PLT	160	165	170	300	150–400

HEMATOLOGY

Specimen	Results				Normal Values
	1/5	1/5	1/6	1/7	
WBC	9.2	9.5	9.8	9.7	4.3–11.0
RBC	4.6	4.8	5.1	5.2	4.5–5.9
HGB	10.1L	10.3L	11.0L	12.1L	13.5–17.5
HCT	44	41	45	44	41–52
MCV	90	89	97	96	80–100
MCHC	44	46	48	50	31–57
PLT	160	165	170	300	150–400

PATIENT X	**ICD-9-CM CODES**
PDX	.
DX2	.
DX3	.
DX4	.
DX5	.
DX6	.
DX7	.
DX8	.
DX9	.
DX10	.

	ICD-9-CM CODES
PP1	.
PR2	.
PR3	.
PR4	.
PR5	.
PR6	.

SAMPLE AMBULATORY CASE

FACE SHEET

DATE OF ADMISSION: 4/5 **DATE OF DISCHARGE:** 4/5

SEX: Male **AGE:** 37 **DISCHARGE DISPOSITION:** Home

ADMISSION DIAGNOSIS: Left inguinal hernia

DISCHARGE DIAGNOSIS: Same

PROCEDURES: Left inguinal herniorrhaphy with excision of lipoma of spermatic cord

HISTORY AND PHYSICAL EXAMINATION

ADMITTED: 4/5

HISTORY OF PRESENT ILLNESS: The patient has been well until several months ago when he began to have pain when lifting.

PAST MEDICAL HISTORY: The patient has no other significant medical or surgical history.

SOCIAL HISTORY: The patient does not use alcohol or tobacco.

ALLERGIES: No known allergies

MEDICATIONS: None

REVIEW OF SYSTEMS:

- **SKIN:** Warm and dry, mucous membranes moist
- **HEENT:** Essentially normal
- **LUNGS:** Clear to percussion and auscultation
- **HEART:** Normal, regular rhythm
- **ABDOMEN:** Normal
- **GENITALIA:** Palpable mass in inguinal canal
- **RECTAL:** Normal
- **EXTREMITIES:** No edema
- **NEUROLOGIC:** Deep tendon reflexes normal

IMPRESSION: Left inguinal hernia

PLAN: Surgical repair of inguinal hernia

PROGRESS NOTES

DATE **NOTE**

4/5 Nursing:

Betadine scrub performed, patient anxious to get surgery over; preoperative medications given as ordered.

4/5 Attending MD:

Brief op note

Dx: Left inguinal hernia

Px: Left inguinal herniorrhaphy

Anes: Local plus sedation

Complications: None

4/5 Attending MD:

No bleeding, patient okay for discharge.

OPERATIVE REPORT

DATE: 4/5

PREOPERATIVE DIAGNOSIS: Left direct inguinal hernia

POSTOPERATIVE DIAGNOSIS: Left direct inguinal hernia

OPERATION: Left inguinal herniorrhaphy

ANESTHESIA: Local plus sedation

OPERATIVE INDICATIONS: A wide mouth direct sac was present in the lower inguinal canal. A lipoma of the cord was present, but no indirect sac.

OPERATIVE PROCEDURE: Under local anesthesia consisting of the equivalent of 19 cc of 1% Xylocaine and 8 cc of _% Marcaine, the abdomen was prepared with Betadine and sterilely draped. A left inguinal incision was made and carried down through subcutaneous tissues to the aponeurosis of the external oblique, which was opened from the external ring to a point over the internal ring. Flaps were cleaned in both directions. The nerve was retracted inferiorly. The cord structures were separated from the surrounding at the level of the pubic tubercle and retracted with a Penrose drain. Cremaster over the cord was opened and a search made for an indirect sac. None was found. Lipoma of the cord was dissected free and clamped at its base and excised. The base was ligated with 00 chromic catgut. Additional cremasteric muscles were divided and ligated with 00 chromic catgut. The direct sac was further dissected down to its base and inverted as the defect was closed by approximating transversus to transversus with a running suture of 00 Vicryl. The floor of the canal was then closed by approximating the internal oblique to the shelving portion of the inguinal ligament with multiple sutures of 0 Ethibond. The external oblique aponeurosis was then reclosed with 0 Ethibond, leaving the cord and nerve in the subcutaneous position. Several sutures of 0 Ethibond were also placed above the emergence of the cord at the internal ring. Subcutaneous tissues were then approximated with 3-0 Vicryl and after irrigation skin was closed with skin clips. The patient tolerated the procedure well and sent to the recovery room in good condition.

PATHOLOGY REPORT

DATE SPECIMEN SUBMITTED: 4/5

SPECIMEN: Lipoma of cord

CLINICAL DATA:

GROSS DESCRIPTION: The specimen is submitted as lipoma of cord. It consists of a single irregularly shaped fragment of fatty tissue that is 8.0 × 4.0 × 1.5 cm. It is covered with a thin membrane.

MICROSCOPIC DESCRIPTION:

DIAGNOSIS: Lipomatous tissue of left spermatic cord

PHYSICIAN'S ORDERS

DATE **ORDER**

4/5 Attending MD:

- Admit to same-day surgery
- Betadine scrub × 3 Pre-op
- May take own meds

4/5 Anesthesia Note:

- Continue NPO
- Demerol 50 mg IM $1^1/_2$ hr Pre-op
- Vistaril 50 mg IM $1^1/_2$ hr Pre-op
- Atropine 0.4 mg IM $1^1/_2$ hr Pre-op

4/5 Attending MD:

- Vital signs q. 15 min until stable
- Regular diet
- Darvocet-N-100 q. 4 hrs p.r.n. pain
- Discharge to home when stable

LABORATORY REPORTS

HEMATOLOGY

DATE: 4/5

Specimen	Results	Normal Values
WBC	6.83	4.3–11.0
RBC	4.57	4.5–5.9
HGB	13.7	13.5–17.5
HCT	43	41–52
MCV	87.0	80–100
MCHC	35	31–57
PLT	300	150–400

AUTO DIFFERENTIAL

Specimen	Results	Normal Values
NEUT	68.3	40.0–74.0
LYMPH	20	19.0–48.0
MONO	5.6	3.4–9.0
EOS	5.6	0.0–7.0
BASO	0.6	0.0–1.5
LUC	3.8	0.0–4.0

URINALYSIS

Test	Result	Ref Range
SP GRAVITY	1.017	1.005–1.035
PH	6	5–7
PROT	TRACE	NEG
GLUC	NONE	NEG
KETONES	NONE	NEG
BILI	NONE	NEG
BLOOD	TRACE	NEG
NITRATES	NONE	NEG
RBCS	NONE	NEG
WBCS	NONE	NEG

RADIOLOGY REPORT

DATE: 4/5

DIAGNOSIS: Inguinal hernia

EXAMINATION: Chest x-ray

Heart size and shape are acceptable. The lung fields are clear and the pulmonary vascular pattern is unremarkable. There is no free fluid and the trachea remains midline.

IMPRESSION: Unremarkable chest x-ray

PATIENT X

PDX

DX2

DX3

DX4

ICD-9-CM CODES

				.		
				.		
				.		
				.		

PP1

PR2

PR3

PR4

PR5

PR6

PR7

CPT CODES

CCS Exam Simulation

In order to simulate the cases that you will need to code, undertake the following:

- Review the list of cases specified here.
- Randomly select 6 inpatient cases and 7 outpatient cases.
- A blank answer sheet is provided at the end of each case.
- Begin to code the 13 cases. *Time yourself so that you remain within the 180 minutes.*
- When all 13 answer sheets have been completed, you will have finished all the cases you need to code.
- Check your answers in the Exam Simulation Answer Key.
- There are more cases than you need to code, so you can get further practice if you need it.

Outpatient Cases

*Refer to ED Mapping Scenario on page 94 to assign E/M codes for ED cases.

Inpatient Cases

Part I: Multiple Choice Questions

A blank answer sheet for these questions can be found on page 71. Please make a copy of this page so that you can record your answers as you go through the questions.

Part I of the CCS examination consists of 60 four-option, multiple choice questions. You will have one hour to complete the multiple choice section during the examination. Please note that you are not permitted to use your codebooks for this section of the examination.

1. A patient is admitted for chest pain and new onset angina was diagnosed. The patient was stabilized and discharged. In a subsequent admission, the patient was admitted as an outpatient for a left heart catheterization, coronary arteriography using two catheters and left ventricular angiography. The patient was found to have arteriosclerotic heart disease. The angina is controlled with medication and the patient has no history of cardiac surgery. The appropriate sequencing of ICD and CPT codes for the outpatient catheterization would be:

411.1	Unstable Angina
413.9	Other and Unspecified Angina Pectoris
414.00	Coronary Arteriosclerosis of Unspecified Type of Vessel, Native or Graft
414.01	Coronary Arteriosclerosis of Native Coronary Artery
786.50	Chest pain
93510	Left heart catheterization
93543	Injection procedure for left ventriculography
93545	Injection procedure for selective angiography
93555	Imaging supervision for left ventricular angiography
93556	Imaging supervision for coronary angiography

   A. 786.50; 93510; 93545; 93555; 93556
   B. 411.1; 93510; 93543; 93545; 93555; 93556
   C. 414.01; 413.9; 93510; 93543; 93545; 93555; 93556
   D. 414.00; 93510; 93543; 93545; 93555; 93556

2. Which of the following is not part of a coding compliance plan?
   A. Regular internal audits
   B. Audits performed by objective external reviewers
   C. Coding audits performed by payers
   D. Sharing and discussing results with coding staff

3. In CPT, unlisted codes are reported only if:
   A. there is not a current CPT category I code available
   B. there is not a current CPT category III code
   C. there is not a current CPT category II code
   D. there is not a current CPT category I or III code

4. A 65-year-old patient is admitted with pain and loosening of a previous total hip arthroplasty. The acetabular component has loosened and become painful. The patient was admitted for revision of the hip replacement. The acetabular component uses a metal-on-metal bearing surface. What would be the appropriate code(s) for the admission?

996.41	Mechanical loosening of prosthetic joint
996.96	Infection and inflammatory reaction to joint prosthesis
V43.64	Organ or tissue replaced by other means
00.71	Revision of hip replacement, acetabular component
00.74	Revision hip replacement bearing surface, metal on polyethylene
00.75	Revision hip replacement bearing surface, metal on metal
00.76	Revision hip replacement bearing surface, ceramic on ceramic

   A. 996.41, V43.64, 00.71, 00.75
   B. 996.96, 00.75
   C. 996.41, V43.64, 00.71
   D. 996.96, V43.64, 00.71, 00.75

5. A 7-year-old patient was admitted to the emergency department for treatment of shortness of breath. The patient is given epinephrine and nebulizer treatments. The shortness of breath and wheezing are unabated following treatment. What diagnosis should be suspected?
   A. Acute bronchitis
   B. Acute bronchitis with chronic obstructive pulmonary disease
   C. Asthma with status asthmaticus
   D. Chronic obstructive asthma

6. Coding policies and procedures can be considered _______ in healthcare organizations.
   A. Organizational tools
   B. Written descriptions of the organization's formal positions
   C. Approved methods for implementing tasks
   D. Guidelines for new coders

7. Under HIPAA Standards for Code Sets, the sets of codes used to encode the diagnoses and procedures, data elements, and medical concepts must be used in _______.
   A. Paper claims only
   B. Electronic claims only
   C. Outpatient claims only
   D. Inpatient claims only

8. A patient is admitted with a high temperature, lethargy, hypotension, tachycardia, oliguria, and elevated WBC. The patient also has more than 100,000 organisms of *Escherichia coli* per cc of urine. The attending physician documents "urosepsis." What is the next step for the coder?
   A. Code sepsis as the principal with a secondary diagnosis of urinary tract infection due to *E coli*
   B. Code urinary tract infection with sepsis as a secondary diagnosis
   C. Query the physician to ask if the patient has septicemia as the patient has the symptomatology
   D. Ask the physician whether the patient had septic shock so that this may be used as the principal diagnosis

9. A virtual screening colonoscopy would be coded as?

45355	Colonoscopy, rigid or flexible, transabdominal via colostomy, single or multiple
45378	Colonoscopy, flexible, proximal to splenic flexure; diagnostic, with or without collection of specimen(s) by brushing or washing, with or without colon decompression (separate procedure)
0066T	Computed tomography (CT) colonography (i.e., virtual colonoscopy); screening
76376	3-D rendering with interpretation and reporting of computed tomography, magnetic resonance imaging, ultrasound, or other tomographic modality, not requiring image postprocessing on an independent workstation

   A. 0066T
   B. 45355
   C. 45378
   D. 76376

Please refer to the following data when answering questions 10 and 11. (Note: The DRG weights are not actual weights for fiscal year 2009.)

MS-DRG	MS-DRG Wt.	Number of Patients
193	3.0	10
195	2.0	10
192	1.0	10

10. The case mix index for the information provided above is:
    A. 0.679
    B. 0.89
    C. 2.0
    D. 0.75

11. The information provided shows that:
    A. The payment is higher for patients with pneumonia with MCCs than without.
    B. There are more patients with pneumonia without MCCs than with MCCs.
    C. There is a large pediatric population at this hospital with pneumonia.
    D. There is inaccurate coding of pneumonia at this institution.

12. If a patient has a principal diagnosis of septicemia, which of the following procedures will increase the DRG assignment the most?
    A. Bronchoscopy with biopsy
    B. Excisional débridement of nails
    C. Excisional débridement of skin ulcer
    D. Ventilator management for greater than 96 hours

13. A maternity patient is admitted in labor at 43 weeks. She has a normal delivery with vacuum extraction to facilitate the baby's delivery. Which of the following would be the principal diagnosis?

650	Normal delivery
645.11	Postterm pregnancy
645.21	Prolonged pregnancy
669.51	Forceps or vacuum delivery without mention of indication

    A. 645.11
    B. 645.21
    C. 650
    D. 669.51

14. Documentation in the record reveals that a patient is admitted with an acute exacerbation of COPD (MS-DRG 192). A higher-paying DRG may be appropriate if documentation is present in the record at the time the decision was made to admit the patient that confirms a diagnosis associated with which of the following:

A. Angina was treated with nitroglycerin prn for chest pain

B. Atrial fibrillation and underwent a cardioversion while hospitalized

C. Blood gases of pO_2 of 58, pCO_2 of 55, pH of 7.32 upon admission and treated with intubation and mechanical ventilation

D. Anemia and was given a blood transfusion

15. A female patient is diagnosed with congestive heart failure. Which of the following will optimize the MS-DRG if it is present?

A. Atrial fibrillation

B. Decubitus ulcer

C. Blood loss anemia

D. Nothing—the DRG does not change if a comorbid condition is added

16. A patient underwent an excision of a benign lesion of the chest that measured 1.0 cm and there was a 0.2 cm margin on both sides. According to the 2009 CPT codes, which code would be used for the procedure?

A. 11401: Excision benign lesion of trunk . . . excised diameter 0.6 cm to 1.0 cm

B. 11601: Excision malignant lesion of trunk . . . excised diameter 0.6 cm to 1.0 cm

C. 11601: Excision malignant lesion of trunk . . . excised diameter 1.1 cm to 2.0 cm

D. 11402: Excision benign lesion of trunk . . . excised diameter 1.1 cm to 2.0 cm

17. If the principal diagnosis is an initial episode of an anterior wall myocardial infarction, which procedure will result in the highest DRG?

A. Mechanical ventilator

B. Insertion central venous catheter

C. Right heart cardiac catheterization

D. Transbronchial lung biopsy

Please use the information in this table to answer questions 18 to 20.

Billing Number	Status Indicator	CPT/HCPCS	APC
989323	V	99285–25	0612
989323	T	25500	0044
989323	X	72050	0261
989323	S	72128	0283
989323	S	70450	0283

18. From the information provided, how many APCs would this patient have?
    A. 1
    B. 5
    C. 4
    D. Unable to determine

19. What percentage will the facility be paid for procedure code 25500?
    A. 50%
    B. 75%
    C. 0%
    D. 100%

20. If another status T procedure were performed, how much would the facility receive for the second status T procedure?
    A. 50%
    B. 75%
    C. 0%
    D. 100%

21. Placenta previa with delivery of twins. This patient had two prior cesarean sections (c-section). She also has a third-degree perineal laceration. This was an emergent c-section due to hemorrhage. The appropriate principal diagnosis would be:
    A. Third-degree perineal laceration
    B. Placenta previa
    C. Twin gestation
    D. Vaginal hemorrhage

22. All of the following are correct **EXCEPT**?
    A. ICD-10-CM and ICD-10-PCS were developed by HHS
    B. NCVHS will hold public hearings before implementation
    C. ICD-10 is already being used in the United States for death certificate coding
    D. The process of adoption of ICD-10-CM is specified in HIPAA

23. A patient is admitted with spotting and fever. She is found to have been treated for a miscarriage with sepsis (which was resolved) two weeks prior to this admission. She is afebrile at this time and is treated with an aspiration dilation and curettage. Products of conception are found. Which of the following should be the principal diagnosis?

    A. Miscarriage

    B. Complications of spontaneous abortion with sepsis

    C. Sepsis

    D. Spontaneous abortion with sepsis

24. A 75-year-old female was admitted for acute myocardial infarction and underwent a diagnostic cardiac catheterization. Following the catheterization, the patient developed a pseudoaneurysm in the common femoral artery. The pseudoaneurysm would be coded as:

    A. 997.2: Peripheral vascular complication and 442.3 other aneurysm of lower extremities

    B. 998.2: Accidental puncture or laceration during a procedure and 442.3 other aneurysm of lower extremities

    C. 442.3: Other aneurysm of artery of lower extremities

    D. 998.2: Accidental puncture or laceration during a procedure

25. A patient was diagnosed with L4-5 lumbar neuropathy and discogenic pain. The patient underwent an intradiscal electrothermal annuloplasty (IDET) in the radiology suite. What ICD-9-CM code should be used?

    A. 80.50: Destruction of intervertebral disc

    B. 04.2: Destruction of cranial and peripheral nerves

    C. 80.59: Other destruction of intervertebral disc

    D. 05.23: Lumbar sympathectomy

26. A patient is admitted with an acute inferior myocardial infarction and discharged alive. Which condition would optimize the DRG?

    A. Respiratory failure

    B. Atrial fibrillation

    C. Hypertension

    D. History of myocardial infarction

27. During a coronary artery bypass surgery, the patient underwent saphenous bypass grafts; from the aorta to the left anterior descending branch of the left main coronary artery, and the left posterior descending of the left main coronary artery. The patient also underwent a repositioning of the mammary artery to the right coronary artery. Please choose the best description for this procedure.

    A. Three (3) aortocoronary grafts

    B. Two (2) aortocoronary grafts and 1 mammary-coronary graft

    C. Two (2) aortocoronary grafts and 2 saphenous bypass graft

    D. Three (3) aortocoronary grafts and 1 mammary-coronary graft

28. A laparoscopic tubal ligation is undertaken. What is the correct CPT code assignment?

49321	Laparoscopy, surgical; with biopsy (single or multiple)
58662	Laparoscopy, surgical; with fulguration or excision of lesions of the ovary, pelvic viscera, or peritoneal surface by any method
58670	Laparoscopy, surgical; with fulguration of oviducts (with or without transection)
58671	Laparoscopy, surgical; with occlusion of oviducts by device (for example, band, clip, or Falope ring)

A. 49321, 58662
B. 58670
C. 58671
D. 49321

29. According to CPT, an endoscopy that is undertaken to the level of the midtransverse colon would be coded as a:

A. Proctosigmoidoscopy
B. Sigmoidoscopy
C. Colonoscopy
D. Proctoscopy

30. Carcinoma of multiple overlapping sites of the bladder. Diagnostic cystoscopy and transurethral fulguration of bladder lesions (1.9 cm, 6.0 cm) are undertaken. The appropriate CPT code(s) would be:

52000	Cystourethroscopy
52224	Cystourethroscopy, with fulguration (including cryosurgery or laser surgery or treatment of minor (less than 0.5 cm) tumor(s) with or without biopsy
52234	Cystourethroscopy, with fulguration (including cryosurgery or laser surgery or treatment of small (less than 0.5 cm to 2.0 cm) tumor(s)
52235	Cystourethroscopy, with fulguration (including cryosurgery or laser surgery or treatment of medium (2.0 cm to 5.0 cm) tumor(s)
52240	Cystourethroscopy, with fulguration (including cryosurgery or laser surgery or treatment of large bladder tumor(s)

A. 52234 and 52240
B. 52235
C. 52240
D. 52000, 52234, 52260

31. According to the AHIMA Standards of Ethical Coding, "A coder should protect the confidentiality of the health record at all times and refuse to access protected health information not required for coding-related activities." Which of the following is not considered a coding-related activity?

    A. Coding audits

    B. Educational purposes within the department

    C. Risk analysis of medical record documentation

    D. Completion of code assignment

32. A patient presents to a facility for upper endoscopy implant of material into the muscle of the lower esophageal sphincter. The correct coding and sequencing of this patient's record is:

    43235 Upper gastrointestinal endoscopy including esophagus, stomach, and either the duodenum and/or jejunum as appropriate; diagnostic, with or without collection of specimen(s) by brushing or washing (separate procedure)

    43257 with delivery of thermal energy to the muscle of lower esophageal sphincter and/or cardia, for treatment of gastroesophageal reflux disease

    43258 with ablation of tumor(s) polyps, or other lesion(s) not amenable to removal by hot biopsy forceps, bipolar cautery or snare technique

    43236 with directed submucosal injection(s), any substance

    A. 43257

    B. 43235, 43236

    C. 43236

    D. 43258, 0133T–50

33. Infusion of Herceptin which is a monoclonal antibody used for treatment of breast cancer in patients carrying a certain mutation of the HER2 gene is classified as _______.

    A. Chemotherapy

    B. Radiotherapy

    C. Genotherapy

    D. Immunotherapy

34. A patient undergoes a colposcopy with endometrial biopsy. Which of the following is correct?

    A. The colposcopy and endometrial biopsy are represented by a combination code

    B. Two codes would be used with modifier –59 appended

    C. Two codes would be used in accordance with 2008 CPT code revisions

    D. Only one code is used and it does not state that it includes endometrial biopsy specifically

35. A patient presents to the outpatient surgical area for a cystoscopy with multiple biopsies of the bladder. The patient's presenting symptom is hematuria. According to the *CPT 2008 Changes: An Insider's View,* what is the correct code assignment for this procedure?

    A. 52000

    B. 52000–22

    C. 52204

    D. 52204–22

36. When a patient receives an injection of IM penicillin G benzathine, 1,000,000 units, what would the appropriate code be to represent the medication?

    90772 Therapeutic, prophylactic or diagnostic injection; subcutaneous or intramuscular

    90774 Therapeutic, prophylactic or diagnostic injection; intravenous push, single or initial

    J0570 Injection, penicillin G benzathine, up to 1,200,000 units

    J0580 Injection, penicillin G benzathine, up to 2,400,000 units

    A. 90782

    B. J0580

    C. 90788

    D. J0570

37. A patient was admitted to the emergency department with chest pain, and was diagnosed with aborted myocardial infarction with acute myocardial ischemia. There was no prior cardiac surgery. The cardiac enzymes were normal. The appropriate coding and sequencing of the diagnosis for this case is:

    A. 410.91: Acute myocardial infarction

    B. 414.01: Arteriosclerotic heart disease or native artery

    C. 411.89: Acute coronary insufficiency

    D. 411.81: Acute coronary occlusion without MI

38. According to the UHDDS, the definition of a secondary diagnosis is a condition that

    A. Is recorded in the patient record

    B. Receives evaluation and is documented by the physician

    C. Receives clinical evaluation, therapeutic treatment, further evaluation, extends the length of stay, increases nursing monitoring/care

    D. Is considered to be essential by the physicians involved and is reflected in the record

39. A patient has nausea and vomiting with abdominal pain due to acute cholecystitis. The physician documents the following on the discharge summary: acute cholecystitis, nausea, vomiting, and abdominal pain. The diagnoses that would be coded are:

    A. Acute cholecystitis, nausea, vomiting, and abdominal pain

    B. Acute cholecystitis, nausea, vomiting

    C. Acute cholecystitis, nausea

    D. Acute cholecystitis

40. The outpatient code editor has all of the following types of edits **EXCEPT**?
    A. Questionable services
    B. Discharge date discrepancy
    C. Service units out of range
    D. Age and procedure edits

41. A patient is admitted because of congestive heart failure (CHF). During the treatment of the CHF the patient was also found to have elevated liver function tests. The physician worked-up the elevated liver function tests but was not able to determine a diagnosis with regard to the abnormal liver tests. The coder should reflect the following diagnosis(es) when coding the record:
    A. Congestive heart failure with liver disease
    B. Abnormal liver function tests
    C. Congestive heart failure and a code from the findings abnormal section
    D. Congestive heart failure

42. A patient is found to have findings suggestive of chronic obstructive pulmonary disease on the chest x-ray. The attending physician mentions the x-ray finding in one progress note but no medication, treatment, or further evaluation is provided. The coder should:
    A. Ask the attending physician if the patient has the condition.
    B. Code the condition because the documentation reflects it.
    C. Question the radiologist regarding whether to code this condition.
    D. Use a code from abnormal findings to reflect the condition.

43. DRG and APC groupers are usually part of an encoding system in which of the following healthcare settings:
    A. Ambulatory surgery centers
    B. Long-term care facilities
    C. Acute care hospitals
    D. Outpatient clinics

44. A patient has an inpatient discharge with principal diagnosis of referred shoulder pain due to peptic ulcer versus cholecystitis. Both are equally treated and well documented. A coder should:
    A. Code whichever diagnosis pays more, if both are equally treated
    B. Use a code from the Findings Abnormal category
    C. Code to the most severe symptom
    D. Code shoulder pain, peptic ulcer, cholecystitis

45. Medical necessity for outpatient services must include all of the following **EXCEPT**:
    A. Medicare number
    B. Physician signature
    C. Diagnosis or signs and symptoms
    D. Service ordered

46. A patient is admitted with hypotension due to dobutamine. How should this be coded?
    A. Orthostatic hypotension 458.0: Adverse effects of dobutamine E941.2
    B. Iatrogenic hypotension, 458.29: Adverse effects of dobutamine E941.2
    C. Other specified hypotension, 458.8: Adverse effects of dobutamine E941.2
    D. Chronic hypotension 458.1: Adverse effects of dobutamine E941.2

47. A patient is undergoing a laparoscopic cholecystectomy. Following the insertion of the laparoscope into the abdominal cavity, the patient experienced a cardiac arrhythmia and the procedure was terminated. The principal procedure would be:
    A. Exploratory laparotomy
    B. Laparoscopy
    C. Laparoscopic removal of the gallbladder
    D. Abdominal paracentesis

48. Data, people, and processes along with a combination of hardware, software, and communications technology are components of a(n) ________.
    A. Information system
    B. Classification system
    C. Operating system
    D. Security information

49. A patient undergoes a laminectomy for spinal stenosis. The patient is readmitted two weeks later for headache and is taken to the operating room to repair a defect in the dura resulting from the laminectomy. The diagnosis or diagnoses for the readmission would be coded as:
    A. 724.02: Spinal stenosis
    B. 998.2: Accidental laceration of dura, 349.0: Spinal fluid loss headache
    C. 952.2: Laceration of dura
    D. 724.02: Spinal stenosis, 952.2: Laceration of the dura

50. A patient was admitted with end stage renal disease with kidney failure following kidney transplant. The patient also had angina and chronic obstructive pulmonary disease. The diagnoses would be coded and sequenced as:
    A. Kidney failure; status post kidney transplant; chronic obstructive pulmonary disease; angina
    B. End stage renal disease; status post kidney transplant; chronic obstructive pulmonary disease; angina
    C. Chronic kidney disease, stage V; status post kidney transplant; chronic obstructive pulmonary disease; angina
    D. Acute Kidney Failure; status post kidney transplant; chronic obstructive pulmonary disease; angina

51. A computer validity check is an example of a control that ensures that data errors do not occur in the first place. This type of control is _______.
    A. Computer
    B. Validity
    C. Maintenance
    D. Preventive

52. If a patient has an excision of a malignant lesion of the skin, the CPT code is determined by the body area from which the excision occurs and the:
    A. Length of the lesion as described in the pathology report
    B. Dimension of the specimen submitted as described in the pathology report
    C. Width times the length of the lesion as described in the operative report
    D. Diameter of the lesion as well as the margins excised as described in the operative report

53. Retention policies for the health information depend on organizational retention policies that must be in accordance with local, state, and federal laws and regulations. These policies vary from institution to institution. In many instances, healthcare institutions may retain health records longer than the law requires. Which of the following statements best describes how the retention of records should be determined?
    A. Unless state or federal law requires longer periods of time, specific patient health information should be retained for established minimum time periods.
    B. AHIMA has published specific guidelines for retention of health information and these guidelines should be followed for records retention.
    C. Joint Commission has developed standards for retention of health information which must be followed to maintain accreditation and these standards should be adhered to according to these guidelines with regard to time frames.
    D. Health records should be retained according to their use in a facility and the state and federal laws do not apply to the retention of this health information.

54. A patient is admitted to the hospital with shortness of breath and congestive heart failure. The patient subsequently develops respiratory failure. The patient undergoes intubation with ventilator management. The correct coding of the case would be:
    A. Congestive heart failure, respiratory failure, ventilator management, intubation
    B. Respiratory failure, intubation, ventilator management
    C. Respiratory failure, congestive heart failure, intubation, ventilator management
    D. Shortness of breath, congestive heart failure, respiratory failure, ventilator management, intubation

55. If a patient is admitted with pneumococcal pneumonia and pneumococcal sepsis, the coder should:
    A. Assign a code for only the sepsis and pneumonia.
    B. Assign a code for the sepsis, pneumonia, and SIRS.
    C. Assign only a code for pneumococcal pneumonia.
    D. Review the chart to determine if septic shock could be used first.

56. A patient is admitted with lethargy, congestive heart failure, and pleural effusion. The patient underwent treatment with diuretics for the CHF, which has cleared. The pleural effusion required a thoracentesis to determine the cause. At the time of discharge the effusion was decreased but not resolved. The correct coding assignment for this case would be:

A. Congestive heart failure

B. Pleural effusion

C. Both congestive heart failure and pleural effusion

D. Lethargy, congestive heart failure, and pleural effusion

57. If a patient undergoes an inpatient procedure and the final summary diagnosis is different from the diagnosis on the pathology report, the coder should:

A. Code only from the discharge diagnoses.

B. Code the diagnosis reflected on the pathology report.

C. Code the most severe symptom.

D. Query the attending physician as to the final diagnosis.

58. Insurance companies are utilizing data warehousing to form clinical repositories by merging their members' claims and clinical data. This information will provide a better understanding of:

A. Cost effectiveness and quality of care

B. Monitoring performance

C. Solving problems

D. Providing feedback to patients

59. A 75-year-old woman is admitted to the hospital after tripping and falling at home. She underwent an open reduction with internal fixation of the femur. Which of the following medications that she takes may indicate a diagnosis that will affect the DRG?

A. Nasabid

B. Lasix

C. Transene

D. Persantine

60. A 56-year-old woman is admitted to an acute care facility from a skilled nursing facility. The patient has multiple sclerosis and hypertension. During the course of hospitalization a decubitus ulcer is found. The ulcer is debrided at the bedside by a physician. There is no typed operative report and no pathology report. The coder should:

A. Use an excisional débridement code as these charts are rarely reviewed to verify the excisional debridement.

B. Code the record with a nonexcisional debridement.

C. Query the physician who performed the debridement to determine if the debridement was excisional.

D. Eliminate the procedure code all together.

Blank Answer Sheet

Use this blank table to fill in your multiple choice answers.

1.	21.	41.
2.	22.	42.
3.	23.	43.
4.	24.	44.
5.	25.	45.
6.	26.	46.
7.	27.	47.
8.	28.	48.
9.	29.	49.
10.	30.	50.
11.	31.	51.
12.	32.	52.
13.	33.	53.
14.	34.	54.
15.	35.	55.
16.	36.	56.
17.	37.	57.
18.	38.	58.
19.	39.	59.
20.	40.	60.

Answers are in the "Exam Simulation Answer Key" section.

Part II: Outpatient Cases

Instructions and official coding guidelines for coding medical records are included in the following resources:

- ICD-9-CM codebook coding conventions, alphabetical and tabular indices
- *ICD-9-CM Official Guidelines* for coding and reporting
- *Coding Clinic for ICD-9-CM* (AHA)
- *Coding Clinic for HCPCS* (AHA)
- Additional coding guidance can be found in the *CPT Assistant* (AMA)

However, hospitals and other organizations may develop their own procedures in the absence of approved guidelines. To ensure consistent coding, the following procedures have been developed for use in the CCS examination. The procedures do not supersede or replace official coding advice and guidelines included in the resources identified above.

These procedures are to be used only in completing the CCS examination. They will be provided to candidates as part of the examination packet. Not adhering to these procedures may result in the miscoding of an exercise, which may result in the deduction of points when the item is scored.

Ambulatory Care Coding

1. Apply ICD-9-CM instructional notations and conventions and current approved "Basic Coding Guidelines for Outpatient Services" and "Diagnostic Coding and Reporting Requirements for Physician Billing" (*Coding Clinic for ICD-9-CM,* 4th Quarter 1995 and 1996) to select diagnoses, conditions, problems, or other reasons for care that require ICD-9-CM coding in an ambulatory care encounter/visit either in a hospital clinic, outpatient surgical area, emergency department, physician's office, or other ambulatory care setting.
2. Sequence the ICD-9-CM code so that the first diagnosis shown in the medical record is the one chiefly responsible for the outpatient services provided during the encounter/visit.
3. Code the secondary diagnoses as follows:
   - A. Chronic diseases that are treated on an ongoing basis may be coded and reported as many times as the patient receives treatment and care for the condition(s).
   - B. Code all documented conditions that coexist at the time of the encounter/visit that require or affect patient care, treatment, or management.
   - C. Conditions previously treated and no longer existing should not be coded.
4. Do not assign External Cause of Injury and Poisoning Codes (E codes), except those that identify the causative substance for an adverse effect of a drug that is correctly prescribed and properly administered (E930–E949).

5. Do not assign Morphology codes (M codes).
6. Do not assign ICD-9-CM procedure codes.
7. Assign CPT codes for all surgical procedures that fall in the surgery section.
8. Assign CPT codes from the following **only if** indicated on the case cover sheet:
    A. Anesthesia section
    B. Medicine section
    C. Evaluation and Management Services section
    D. Radiology section
    E. Laboratory and Pathology section
9. Assign CPT/HCPCS modifiers for hospital-based facilities, if applicable (regardless of payer).
10. Do not assign HCPCS Level II (alphanumeric) codes.

The CCS Examination is an intimidating task but tackle one patient record at a time. You have to code a total of 13 records—6 inpatient records and 7 outpatient records. Randomly select the cases—6 inpatient and 7 outpatient—to simulate the examination.

Answers and references for the cases are provided in the Exam Simulation Answer Key.

SAME DAY SURGERY SUMMARY—Patient 1

HISTORY AND PHYSICAL EXAMINATION—Patient 1

REASON FOR ADMISSION: Breast mass

HISTORY OF PRESENT ILLNESS: The patient is a 57-year-old woman who had a routine mammogram performed last week. A lump was noted on the mammogram about 1.2 cm. in size. The patient was referred to me. After an explanation to the patient about the condition, a needle localization breast biopsy was performed which revealed ductal carcinoma in situ.

PAST MEDICAL HISTORY: Noncontributory

ALLERGIES: None known

CHRONIC MEDICATIONS: None

SOCIAL HISTORY: The patient is a 57-year-old female who is married and lives with her husband. She is a nondrinker and a nonsmoker.

REVIEW OF SYSTEMS: The patient has normal bowels. There is no hematuria or dysuria. The patient has had two colds in the past six weeks. She states that she has been having some difficulty sleeping because of worry over this beast mass.

PHYSICAL EXAMINATION: This is a well-developed, well-nourished 57-year-old female who appears younger than her stated age.

HEENT: PERRLA with supple neck

Lungs: The lungs are clear to percussion and auscultation

Chest: The heart has normal rhythm and pulse. There is a mass in the right breast

Abdomen: Abdomen reveals no masses; bowel sounds are heard

Extremities: Extremities reveal no edema

IMPRESSION: Ductal carcinoma right breast

PLAN: The patient came back to the office yesterday morning with her husband. The situation was explained to them. Since this is a ductal carcinoma in situ. Lumnectomy will be performed and sentinel node dissection will be carried out. Whether the patient needs further treatment or not depends on the findings of the permanent sections of the specimen. The patient and her husband understand the situation very well and agreed to proceed with surgery.

OPERATIVE REPORT—Patient 1

PREOPERATIVE DIAGNOSIS: Ductal carcinoma in situ, right breast, status post biopsy.

POSTOPERATIVE DIAGNOSIS: Ductal carcinoma in situ, right breast, status post biopsy.

OPERATION: Lumpectomy and sentinel axillary lymph node dissection.

ANESTHESIA: General anesthesia with laryngeal intubation

PROCEDURE: After obtaining the informed consent, the patient was brought into the operating room and placed on the table in the supine position. General anesthesia with laryngeal intubation was conducted smoothly. The skin over the right chest and right arm was prepped and draped in the usual sterile manner. The intended incision line was marked with a marking pen. The blue dye for the sentinel node dissection was injected. The breast tissue was massaged. Five minutes were then allowed to pass before the incision was made.

The incision was made with excision of the previous incisional scar. The lymphatics were identified and dissected. The suspicious axillary sentinel nodes were dissected. Then the lumpectomy was performed with upper and lower skin flaps. The dissection of the breast tissue and subcutaneous tissue to raise the two flaps was conducted smoothly. A large lump was dissected and the dissection carried to the pectoralis muscles. The big lump was removed completely. Hemostasis was confirmed by cauterization. The wound was then irrigated with copious amounts of warm water solution. The specimen was sent to pathology and the sentinel nodes were sent separately to pathology. The wound was then closed in layers using 2-0 Vicryl for the deeper layer, 3-0 Vicryl for the subcutaneous tissue, and 4-0 Vicryl for the skin.

The patient tolerated the whole procedure very well and was sent to the recovery room in stable condition after extubation.

Blood loss was minimal. Sponge and needle counts were correct. No drain was left. The specimens were sent to pathology.

PATHOLOGY REPORT—Patient 1

DATE: 8/3

SPECIMEN: Breast lump and lymph node

GROSS DESCRIPTION: The specimen is submitted as breast and lymphatic tissue. It consists of breast tissue measuring 2.0 cm, 1.5 cm, 1.0 cm.

DIAGNOSIS: Ductal carcinoma insitu

PATIENT 1

ICD-9-CM CODES

PDX					.		
DX2					.		
DX3					.		
DX4					.		

CPT CODES

PP1					
PR2					
PR3					
PR4					
PR5					
PR6					
PR7					

SAME DAY SURGERY SUMMARY—Patient 2

DATE OF ADMISSION: 8/3 **DATE OF DISCHARGE**: 8/3

DISCHARGE DIAGNOSIS:

1. Sinus infection
2. Chronic otitis media
3. Adenoid hypertrophy

PROCEDURES:

1. Adenoidectomy
2. Bilateral myringotomy

INSTRUCTIONS ON DISCHARGE:

Contact my office for follow-up in one week
Take Augmentin 500 mg by mouth BID per day for 10 days
Darvocet 1 tablet every 4 hours for pain as needed

HISTORY AND PHYSICAL EXAMINATION—Patient 2

ADMITTED: 8/3

REASON FOR ADMISSION: This is a 35-year-old patient who has recurrent sinusitis and chronic otitis media. The patient also suffers from adenoidal obstruction of the eustachian tubes and nasopharynx. Treatment has consisted of antihistamines and decongestants as well as antibiotic therapy. This has been ineffective to control the inflammation. The patient has requested surgery for definitive treatment of the condition.

PAST MEDICAL HISTORY: Negative

ALLERGIES: None known

CHRONIC MEDICATIONS: None

FAMILY HISTORY: Noncontributory

REVIEW OF SYSTEMS: The patient has had repeated office visits over the past three years for sinusitis and otitis media. The patient has no other health problems.

PHYSICAL EXAMINATION: This is a Hispanic female in no acute distress. BP is 120/70. Temp. is 99.0 degrees. Pulse is 72. Respirations 12.

HEENT: Tympanic membranes are red with perforation of the tympanic membrane and hearing loss. Otherwise normal.

NECK: Supple

CHEST: Clear to percussion and auscultation

HEART: Regular force, rate, and rhythm

ABDOMINAL: Normal, no masses

EXTREMITIES: No edema, normal

IMPRESSION: Sinus infection and chronic otitis media

PROGRESS NOTES—Patient 2

DATE NOTE

8/3 Patient is alert and oriented. Admitted to Same Day Surgery for adenoidectomy and insertion of myringotomy tubes.

Preoperative diagnosis:
Chronic sinusitis

Postoperative diagnosis:

1. Chronic sinusitis
2. Otitis media; Adenoid obstruction of the eustachian tube and nasopharynx

Operation:
Bilateral myringotomy with insertion of Shepard tympanostomy tubes;
Adenoidectomy

Anesthesia: General
Complications: None

The patient tolerated the procedure well. No bleeding noted. Will discharge patient when transportation available.

PHYSICIAN'S ORDERS—Patient 2

DATE ORDER

8/3 The patient is admitted for adenoidectomy and myringotomy.
Prep patient for surgery
NPO
PRE OP Orders
Morphine 10 mg IM upon admission
Atropine 0.4 mg IM upon admission

Post-op Orders
Ice collar
T & A Precautions
OOB ad lib
Darvocet-N tabs, one every 4 hours p.r.n. pain
Demerol 75 mg. PO now

Discharge after 4:00 p.m. when stable

OPERATIVE REPORT—Patient 2

DATE: 8/3

PREOPERATIVE DIAGNOSIS: Chronic sinusitis, otitis media, adenoid obstruction of the eustachian tubes and nasopharynx

POSTOPERATIVE DIAGNOSIS: Chronic sinusitis, serous otitis media, adenoid obstruction of the eustachian tubes and nasopharynx

OPERATION: Bilateral myringotomy with insertion of Shepard tympanostomy tubes; Adenoidectomy

ANESTHESIA: General

OPERATIVE PROCEDURE: Following the induction of general anesthesia, the patient was prepped and draped in the usual sterile manner for the above mentioned procedures. The left ear was approached first.

The tympanic membrane was found to be injected, retracted, and full of a serous fluid. An anterior myringotomy incision was performed, and a Shepard tympanostomy tube was inserted in place.

Following this, an identical procedure was done on the right side, except on the right side the fluid was gray and viscous, and the tympanic membrane had already developed tympanosclerotic scar tissue throughout the tympanic membrane. An anterior myringotomy incision was performed, and a Shepard tympanostomy tube was inserted in place.

Following this, the patient was prepared and draped in the usual manner for adenoidectomy. With the soft palate retracted, an adenoid mass filling the entire nasopharynx was visualized. It was removed with adenoid curets until the normal anatomical structures of the torus tubarius and the posterior choanae of the nasal passages could clearly be seen. The adenoid tissue trailed into the nose and into the area of the infundibulum of the middle meatus. Hemostasis was achieved.

The patient was awakened from anesthesia and taken to the recovery room in good condition.

PATHOLOGY REPORT—Patient 2

DATE: 8/3

SPECIMEN: Adenoids

GROSS DESCRIPTION: The specimen is submitted as adenoids. It consists of multiple fragments of adenoid tissue, the largest measuring 2.5 cm, 1.5 cm, 1.0 cm. These fragments are similar to tonsillar tissues. There are no significant pathologic lesions seen grossly.

MICROSCOPIC DESCRIPTION:

DIAGNOSIS: Adenoids

PATIENT 2

ICD-9-CM CODES

PDX					.		
DX2					.		
DX3					.		
DX4					.		

CPT CODES

PP1					
PR2					
PR3					
PR4					
PR5					
PR6					
PR7					

SAME DAY SURGERY SUMMARY—PATIENT 3

HISTORY AND PHYSICAL EXAMINATION—Patient 3

DATE: 1/29

HISTORY OF PRESENT ILLNESS: This is a 62-year-old gentleman with progressive painful blurring of vision due to aphakic bullous keratopathy with glaucoma. He has undergone previous Molteno implant with poor vision and pain due to ruptured bulla. The patient is admitted for transplant vitrectomy and lens implantation at this time.

PAST MEDICAL HISTORY: The patient has angina and COPD. There have been no recent episodes of chest pain or shortness of breath. The patient also underwent a prostatectomy six years ago for prostatic carcinoma.

ALLERGIES: None known

CHRONIC MEDICATIONS: Ventolin and nitroglycerin as needed for chest pain

SOCIAL HISTORY: The patient is a 62-year-old male who is married and lives with his wife. He has 5 grandchildren. He is a nondrinker and a nonsmoker.

REVIEW OF SYSTEMS: The patient had normal bowels. He has had no problems with his urine since his prostatectomy. There is no hematuria or dysuria. The patient has had two colds in the past six weeks. He states that he has been having some difficulty sleeping because of the pain in his shoulder. This has limited some of the activity that he normally does, such as golf.

PHYSICAL EXAMINATION: This is a well-developed, well-nourished 62-year-old male who appears younger than his stated age.

HEENT: Aphakic, neck supple

Chest: The lungs are clear to percussion and auscultation. The heart has normal rhythm and pulse

Abdomen: Abdomen reveals no masses; bowel sounds are heard

Extremities: Extremities reveal no edema

OPERATIVE REPORT—Patient 3

PREOPERATIVE DIAGNOSES:
1. Aphakic bullous keratopathy
2. Open-angle glaucoma
3. Chronic iritis

POSTOPERATIVE DIAGNOSES:
1. Aphakic bullous keratopathy
2. Open-angle glaucoma
3. Chronic iritis

OPERATION:
1. Aphakic penetrating keratoplasty
2. Posterior chamber intraocular lens scleral implant
3. Open-sky mechanical automated vitrectomy

ANESTHESIA: Retrobulbar block, monitored anesthesia care

COMPLICATIONS: None

INDICATIONS: This is a 62-year-old gentleman with progressive painful blurring of vision due to aphakic bullous keratopathy with glaucoma. He has undergone previous Molteno implant with poor vision and pain due to ruptured bulla. The patient is admitted for transplant vitrectomy and lens implantation of the left eye at this time. After informed consent, the patient agreed to the benefits and risks of surgery.

PROCEDURE DESCRIPTION:

The patient was taken to the operating room. Under monitored anesthesia care, he was given a retrobulbar block in the standard fashion for a total of 4 cc of a 50/50 mixture 0.75% Marcaine and 4% lidocaine with Wydase.

After ensuring adequate anesthesia as well as akinesia, the patient was prepped and draped in the usual sterile ophthalmologic fashion. A wire lid speculum was inserted, and a small conjunctival peritomy was made at the two o'clock and ten o'clock hour positions to prepare for half-thickness scleral flaps for suturing a scleral-supported lens in the left eye. A Flieringa ring was then attached in the standard fashion using four interrupted 5-0 Dacron sutures. Attention was then placed to the back Mayo, and a 7.75-mm donor button was harvested, epithelial side down, in the standard fashion. Routine surveillance cultures were sent, and the donor button was placed on the Mayo stand in a Petri dish. Attention was then placed on the donor's cornea, and using a Barron-Hessburg trephine device, a 7.50-mm button was harvested under viscoelastic support. Corneoscleral scissors were used to the left and right respectively to remove the button in toto. Vitrectomy was then performed due to prolapsing vitreous, and an attempt to reposition the iris was made. However, due to loss of iris material during prior surgeries, I was unable to close the sphincter defect. After completing the vitrectomy, a scleralsupported CZ70VD 7-mm lens was secured using a 10-0 Prolene suture at the ten and two o'clock hour positions. Scleral flaps were then closed over the 10-0 Prolene to maintain a tight closure. The button was then sewn into pos ion using 16 interrupted 10-0 nylon sutures in the standard fashion. All the knots were cut short and buried in the recipient side of the host junction. A final check to make sure the chamber was watertight was unremarkable, and the Flieringa ring was removed followed by the bridle sutures. Subconjunctival Ancef and Celestone were placed, and a bandage contact lens was placed on the eye.

The patient was taken to the recovery room in good repair without complications of the above procedure.

PATIENT 3

PDX

DX2

DX3

DX4

ICD-9-CM CODES

CPT CODES

PP1

PR2

PR3

PR4

PR5

PR6

PR7

SAME DAY SURGERY RECORD—Patient 4

DATE OF ADMISSION: 1/29 **DATE OF DISCHARGE**: 1/29

DISCHARGE DIAGNOSIS Torn lateral meniscus of the right knee; torn anterior cruciate ligament of the right knee

ADMISSION HISTORY: The patient is a 17-year-old male who approximately 1 year ago underwent a cruciate ligament reconstruction. He has had several reinjuries and for this reason was taken for arthroscopic evaluation and treatment.

COURSE IN HOSPITAL: The patient was taken to the OR where a resection of tear of the lateral meniscus posterior horn and reconstruction of the anterior cruciate ligament using patellar tendon graft was performed. The patient was then discharged and asked to return in 1 week.

INSTRUCTIONS ON DISCHARGE:

Levaquin 500 mg by mouth, 1 per day
Tylox 1–2 capsules as needed for pain
Follow-up appointment in 1 week

HISTORY AND PHYSICAL EXAMINATION—Patient 4

DATE: 1/29

HISTORY OF PRESENT ILLNESS: This is a 17-year-old male active in several sports. He then reinjured the knee several times this year while playing soccer.

PAST MEDICAL HISTORY: The patient has no other health problems.

ALLERGIES: None known

CHRONIC MEDICATIONS: None

FAMILY HISTORY: Noncontributory

PHYSICAL EXAMINATION: Reveals a well-developed, well-nourished white male in no apparent distress. HEENT reveals nothing abnormal. Chest was clear to auscultation and percussion. Heart sounds were normal with no murmurs. Examination of the abdomen reveals no masses or tenderness. Examination of the genitals was not done. Examination of the extremities reveals a scar on the left knee with swelling of the joint. Distal sensation and circulation were normal.

IMPRESSION: Torn lateral meniscus of the right knee; torn anterior cruciate ligament of the right knee.

PLAN:
1. Resection of tear of the lateral meniscus posterior horn.
2. Reconstruction of the anterior cruciate ligament using patellar tendon graft

PROGRESS NOTES—Patient 4

DATE	NOTE
1/29	Admit to Same Day Surgery Unit Prep for surgery Betadine scrub right leg Demerol 100 mg IM 1 hr preop Versed 5 mg IM 1 hr preop Postop Orders: Demerol 75 mg. PRN pain 1 dose Tylox 1 to 2 PO q. 4 hr Levaquin 500 mg PO postop D/C when stable as per discharge criteria

PHYSICIAN'S ORDERS—Patient 4

DATE	ORDER
1/29	Patient admitted for surgical and diagnostic arthroscopy. OP-note PREOP DX: Torn lateral meniscus of the right knee; torn anterior cruciate ligament of the right knee. POSTOP DX: Torn lateral meniscus of the right knee; torn anterior cruciate ligament of the right knee.

OPERATION:
1. Resection of tear of the lateral meniscus posterior horn.
2. Reconstruction of the anterior cruciate ligament using patellar tendon graft

ANES: General
Good circulation and sensation. Will encourage patient to ambulate with splint and crutches. Discharge when stable. Follow-up in one week with my office.

DISCHARGE MEDICATIONS:
Levaquin 500 mg by mouth, one per day
Tylox 1–2 capsules as needed for pain

OPERATIVE REPORT—Patient 4

PREOPERATIVE DIAGNOSIS: Torn lateral meniscus of the right knee; torn anterior cruciate ligament of the right knee

POSTOPERATIVE DIAGNOSIS: Torn lateral meniscus of the right knee; torn anterior cruciate ligament of the right knee

OPERATION:
1. Resection of tear of the lateral meniscus posterior horn
2. Reconstruction of the anterior cruciate ligament using patellar tendon graft

ANESTHESIA: General

CLINICAL HISTORY: This is a 17-year-old male who sustained an injury to his right knee in May during a surfing accident. He was treated conservatively before this. But because of instability and pain, he wished to have the following procedure done.

Tourniquet was used for one hour, 50 minutes

PROCEDURE DESCRIPTION: The patient was placed under general anesthesia. Airway was maintained by Dr. Spears, as the right lower limb was manipulated and found to have a positive Lachman, a positive drawer test, and a trace pivot shift. The left knee was also examined and found to have the same findings.

The knee was prepped with a gel prep, draped with the limb free. Tourniquet was applied to the thigh but not elevated to begin with. The procedure done first was a diagnostic arthroscopy and during this, we found that the anterior cruciate ligament was torn away from the wall lateral femoral condyle. It was quite lax as well. Attention was turned to the lateral compartment where the initial look at the lateral cartilage showed that it was fine. But on probing underneath the surface of the posterior horn, there was a partial tear but without any instability. The tear extended through the cartilage 50 to 75%. Because of this, this portion was resected back to normal cartilage, removing the torn segment. This was in an area that was not vascular.

Attention was then turned to the anterior cruciate ligament which was resected. Using a shaver, all the soft tissue was removed from around and up into the notch. A bur was used to enlarge the notch superiorly, into the lateral side and into the depth of the notch to the over-the-top position which was clearly delineated.

The first part of the arthroscopy was terminated. The tourniquet was elevated. Then an incision was made from the mid patella to the tibial tubercle, with dissection carried down to the patellar tendon. The middle third of the patellar tendon was harvested with bone graft from tibia and fibula which was sized to a 10-rom tunnel size. Two threads were placed in the femoral portion and one in the tibial portion, and the femoral portion marked at the interface between the bone and the tendon. The small saw was used to cut the bone graft from both the tibia and the patella. The patellar defect was filled with bone graft and closed. The guide for the tibial tunnel was then put in place, measuring about 55 degrees. This was placed just in front of the posterior tibial tendon and in the mid portion of the slope of the tibial spine. The guide wire was put in place, found to be satisfactory, and a 10-rom channel was reamed. The over-thetop positioning was put into placed with a guidewire. This was in the eleven o'clock for the right knee. The bulldog cannulated reamer was used, and a footprint was established. Probing revealed there to be a millimeter of bone posterior to this. This was reamed up to 30 mm in size for the graft plus 5 rom. The guidewire was removed. The eccentric guide was put into place, and a notch made. Then the two-pin passer was passed through the eccentric guide, and then the guide was removed. The exit of the two-pin passer was in a proper place on the anterolateral thigh. A guidewire was used to put in place in the two-pin passer, and the gra was passed up into the channel and seemed to fit well. A biodegradable screw was used, but the rst one did not cut properly and had to be replaced after tapping the spot for the screw. A second biodegradable screw was put up in place. This was approximately 25 × 9 mm. The position and tightness were excellent, and drawer test at this point was trace, as was the Lachman. There was no impingement of the graft with extension, and no change in the length. The screw for the tibia was put into place over a guidewire, and this was an 8 × 25 tibial screw. This again was quite tight, and the Lachman test was just a trace positive.

The joint and the wound were irrigated with arthroscopic fluid, and subcutaneous tissues were closed with 2-0 Vicryl. The skin was closed with 4-0 nylon, as was each of the ports. The incision plus the ports were all injected with 0.25% Marcaine with epinephrine. The patient was given 30 mg of Toradol. Dressing was applied of Xeroform gauze, 4 × 4s, Kerlix, Ace wrap, and then the patient's brace which was a Bledsoe brace.

He tolerated the procedure well with a tourniquet time of 1 hour 50 minutes. Blood loss was nil. He will be sent home on Lortab. He will return to the office on Friday for a dressing change. He will be contacted tomorrow.

PHYSICIAN'S ORDERS—Patient 4

DATE	**ORDER**
4/1/200X	Attending MD: Admit to same-day surgery Betadine scrub × 3 Preop May take own meds Lasix 20 mg now
4/1/200X	Anesthesia Note: Continue NPO Demerol 50 mg IM 1½ hr Preop Vistaril 50 mg IM 1½ hr Preop Atropine 0.4 mg IM 1½ hr Preop
4/1/200X	Attending MD: Vital signs q. 15 min until stable Regular diet Darvocet-N-100 q. 4 hrs p.r.n. pain Iron supplement q.d. for anemia Discharge to home when stable

LABORATORY REPORTS—Patient 4

HEMATOLOGY

DATE: 3/31

Specimen	Results	Normal Values
WBC	7.2	4.3–11.0
RBC	4.0 L	4.5–5.9
HGB	11.0 L	13.5–17.5
HCT	38.0 L	41–52
MCV	94	80–100
MCHC	40	31–57
PLT	300	150–400

PATIENT 4

ICD-9-CM CODES

PDX

DX2

DX3

DX4

CPT CODES

PP1

PR2

PR3

PR4

PR5

PR6

PR7

SAME DAY SURGERY SUMMARY—Patient 5

DATE OF ADMISSION: 12/30 **DATE OF DISCHARGE**: 12/30

DISCHARGE DIAGNOSIS: Bunion with hypertrophy of 1st metatarsal

ADMISSION HISTORY: This is a 45-year-old white female in good health. Her family physician has performed a history and physical that demonstrated her health is within normal limits. The patient has no known allergies, good pedal pulses. The patient has a bunion of the left 1st metatarsal causing hypertrophy.

COURSE IN HOSPITAL: The patient was admitted to same-day surgery for osteotomy of the 1st metatarsal for hypertrophy. The patient was taken to the OR where this was accomplished. The patient tolerated the procedure well and is discharged to home in stable condition.

INSTRUCTIONS ON DISCHARGE:

Keep foot elevated.
Keep dressing dry; do not change until seen by your physician.
Use surgical shoe.
Take Darvocet N 100 mg every 4 hours as needed for pain.

HISTORY AND PHYSICAL EXAMINATION—Patient 5

DATE: 12/30

HISTORY OF PRESENT ILLNESS: The patient has had increased long-term pain with difficulty ambulating.

PAST MEDICAL HISTORY: The patient has no major health problems and has not undergone major surgery.

ALLERGIES: None known

CHRONIC MEDICATIONS: None

FAMILY HISTORY: Noncontributory

PHYSICAL EXAMINATION:

IMPRESSION: B.P. 130/88, pulse is 68, respirations 20, temp 97.3. HEENT, within normal limits. Heart, normal. Lungs, clear. Abdomen, soft with bowel sounds. Pelvic and rectal deferred. Extremities, normal except bunion on 1st metatarsal.

PLAN: Osteotomy with excision of 1st metatarsal eminence

PROGRESS NOTES—Patient 5

DATE **NOTE**

12/30 This is a 45-year-old female admitted for ostectomy to relieve long-term pain in the left foot. The patient is good health.
D/C when stable as per discharge criteria

Patient admitted for surgery
OP-NOTE:
PREOP DX: Bunion with hypertrophy of 1st metatarsal
POSTOP DX: Same
OPERATION: Osteotomy with excision of 1st metatarsal eminence
ANES: Digital
Good circulation and sensation. Will encourage patient to ambulate with splint and crutches

Discharge when stable. Follow-up in one week with my office.
Discharge Medications: None

PHYSICIAN'S ORDERS—Patient 5

DATE **ORDER**

12/30 Admit to Same-Day Surgery Unit
Prep for surgery
Vistaril 50 mg PO 1 hour preop
Atropine 0.8 mg PO 1 hour preop

Post-op orders:
Continue to elevate foot
Darvocet N 100 mg every 4 hours p.r.n. pain
Discharge patient when surgical shoe procured

OPERATIVE REPORT—Patient 5

DATE: 12/30

PREOPERATIVE DIAGNOSIS: Hypertrophy of the 1st left metatarsal head

POSTOPERATIVE DIAGNOSIS: Same

OPERATION: Osteotomy with partial excision of the 1st left metatarsal head

ANESTHESIA: Digital

OPERATIVE PROCEDURE:

With the patient under local standby anesthesia and in the supine position she was properly prepped and draped. The tourniquet was applied about the left ankle superior to the malleoli.

A lazy "S" type incision was made on the lateral side of the 1st metatarsal head. This incision was deepened by blunt and sharp dissection until the capsule of the 1st metatarsophalangeal joint, left was reached. A linear incision measuring approximately 4 cm in length was made. Approximately 0.5 cm of bone was removed from the medial aspect of the 1st metatarsal head with oscillating saw. An osteotomy through the neck of the same bone was undertaken with an osteotome. Following alignment of bone, a wire link was placed. The joint capsule was closed with continuous suture of 2-0 chromic catgut and the subcutaneous tissue was closed with continuous suture of 4-0 chromic catgut and the skin was closed with continuous suture of 4-0 nylon.

The wound was dressed with Vaseline gauze and gentle fluff pressure dressing. The patient was discharged from the operating suite in good condition noting that vascularity had returned to all five toes.

PATHOLOGY REPORT—Patient 5

DATE: 12/30

SPECIMEN: Bunion from the 1st toe left foot

GROSS DESCRIPTION: The specimen consists of a dome-shaped fragment of hypertrophic osseous tissue that measures 1.2 × 1.1 × 0.5 cm. Decalcification.

MICROSCOPIC DESCRIPTION: Sections of the decalcified tissue reveal fragments of hypertrophic osteocartilagenous tissue. No evidence of metastatic disease or neutrophilic inflammatory infiltrate was noted.

DIAGNOSIS: Bone (left 1st toe): Fragments of hypertrophic osteocartilagenous tissue

PATIENT 5

ICD-9-CM CODES

PDX

DX2

DX3

DX4

				.		
				.		
				.		
				.		

CPT CODES

PP1

PR2

PR3

PR4

PR5

PR6

PR7

Emergency Department (ED) Evaluation and Management (E/M) Mapping Scenario for Emergency Department Cases 6 to 8*

Code the procedures that are done in the ED as well as the E/M code derived from the E/M Mapping Scenario.

Point Value Key

Level 1 = 1–20

Level 2 = 21–35

Level 3 = 36–47

Level 4 = 48–60

Level 5 = ≥ 61

Critical Care ≥ 61 with constant physician attendance

CPT Codes

Level 1	99281	99281–25 with procedure/laboratory/radiology
Level 2	99282	99282–25 with procedure/laboratory/radiology
Level 3	99283	99283–25 with procedure/laboratory/radiology
Level 4	99284	99284–25 with procedure/laboratory/radiology
Level 5	99285	99285–25 with procedure/laboratory/radiology

Emergency Department Acuity Points

	5	**10**	**15**	**20**	**25**
Meds Given	1–2	3–5	6–7	8–9	> 10
Extent of Hx	Brief	PF	EPF	Detail	Comprehensive
Extent of Examination	Brief	PF	EPF	Detail	Comprehensive
# of Tests Ordered	0–1	2–3	4–5	6–7	> 8
Supplies Used	1	2–3	4–5	6–7	> 8

EMERGENCY DEPARTMENT RECORD—Patient 6

DATE OF ADMISSION: 4/1 **DATE OF DISCHARGE**: 4/1

HISTORY (Problem Focused):

HISTORY OF PRESENT ILLNESS: This 16-year-old black female underwent piercing of her ears. The patient was removing her sweater when she accidentally pulled the earring through her ear lobe.

PAST MEDICAL HISTORY: The patient has a history of childhood asthma that has not occurred for several years.

ALLERGIES: Penicillin

CHRONIC MEDICATIONS: None

REVIEW OF SYSTEMS: The patient has been well.

PHYSICAL EXAMINATION (Problem Focused):

GENERAL APPEARANCE: This is a well-nourished 16-year-old black female in no apparent distress. HEENT normal except for 2 cm laceration of left earlobe. Neck veins flat at 40-degree angle. No nodes felt in the neck, carotids, or groin. Carotid pulsations are normal. No bruits heard in the neck. Chest clear on percussion and auscultation. Heart is not enlarged. No thrills or murmurs. Rhythm is regular. BP 130/80. Liver and spleen not palpable. No masses felt in the abdomen. No ascites noted. No edema of the extremities. Pulses in the feet are good.

IMPRESSION: Laceration of left ear lobe

PLAN: Suture laceration of ear lobe

TREATMENT: Following infiltration of the areas with Xylocaine, the laceration was closed with 2-0 Vicryl. Two suture kits were used.

DISCHARGE DIAGNOSIS: Ear lobe laceration of left ear

INSTRUCTIONS ON DISCHARGE: Demerol by mouth 50 mg every 6 hours as needed for pain. Biaxin 500 mg PO b.i.d. for 10 days. Follow-up with surgical clinic in 7 days.

PATIENT 6

ICD-9-CM CODES

PDX						
DX2						
DX3						
DX4						

CPT CODES

PP1					
PR2					
PR3					
PR4					
PR5					
PR6					
PR7					

EMERGENCY DEPARTMENT RECORD—Patient 7

DATE OF ADMISSION: 6/17 **DATE OF DISCHARGE**: 6/17

HISTORY (Problem Focused):

ADMISSION HISTORY: This is a 29-year-old Asian female. She was walking down her steps when she fell. The patient complains of pain in the arm.

ALLERGIES: Penicillin

CHRONIC MEDICATIONS: Normally takes no drugs but has been taking ibuprofen every 6 hours because of painful arm.

FAMILY HISTORY: Noncontributory

SOCIAL HISTORY: The patient smokes one pack of cigarettes per day. She drinks one drink per day.

REVIEW OF SYSTEMS: The patient had hives the last time she took penicillin. Her cardiovascular, genitourinary, and gastrointestinal systems are negative.

PHYSICAL EXAMINATION (Expanded Problem Focused):

GENERAL APPEARANCE: This is an alert cooperative female in no acute distress.

HEENT: PERRLA, extraocular movements are full

NECK: Supple

CHEST: Lungs are clear. Heart has normal sinus rhythm.

ABDOMEN: Soft and nontender, no organomegaly

EXTREMITIES: Examination of the arm reveals painful movement

LABORATORY AND X-RAY DATA: Urinalysis is normal, EKG normal, chest x-ray is normal. CBC and diff show no abnormalities. X-ray of the left arm revealed a fracture of the shaft of the humerus.

IMPRESSION: Fracture of the shaft of the humerus

PLAN: Reduction fracture of the humerus

TREATMENT: Following administration of conscious sedation, the patient's humeral fracture was reduced and a cast applied. One fracture tray was used.

DISCHARGE DIAGNOSIS: Fracture of the left shaft of the humerus.

INSTRUCTIONS ON DISCHARGE: The patient is instructed to make an appointment with the orthopedic clinic in 3 days, to take one Percocet every 4 hours as needed for pain as per the label. Call the ER doctor if swelling or blue color of the fingers occurs.

PATIENT 7

PDX

DX2

DX3

DX4

ICD-9-CM CODES

				.		
				.		
				.		
				.		

PP1

PR2

PR3

PR4

PR5

PR6

PR7

CPT CODES

EMERGENCY DEPARTMENT RECORD—Patient 8

DATE OF ADMISSION: 8/19 **DATE OF DISCHARGE**: 8/19

HISTORY (Problem Focused):

ADMISSION HISTORY: This is a 13-year-old African-American male. He became short of breath, used his inhaler as described but continued to have wheezing and short of breath.

ALLERGIES: None

CHRONIC MEDICATIONS: Albuterol inhaler

FAMILY HISTORY: Noncontributory

SOCIAL HISTORY: The patient's father smokes one pack of cigarettes per day but he does not smoke in the house.

REVIEW OF SYSTEMS: His integumentary, musculoskeletal, cardiovascular, genitourinary, and gastrointestinal systems are negative.

PHYSICAL EXAMINATION (Extended Problem Focused):

GENERAL APPEARANCE: This is an alert, cooperative young male in acute distress.

HEENT: PERRLA, extraocular movements are full

NECK: Supple

CHEST: Lungs reveal wheezes and rales. Heart has normal sinus rhythm.

ABDOMEN: Soft and nontender, no organomegaly

EXTREMITIES: Examination is normal

LABORATORY DATA: Urinalysis is normal, EKG normal, chest x-ray is normal. CBC and diff show no abnormalities.

IMPRESSION: Acute asthma with exacerbation

PLAN: Administer epinephrine and intravenous theophylline

TREATMENT: Following administration of epinephrine and theophylline, the patient's asthma abated. One venipuncture set and one IV set were used to administer the medication over 30 minutes.

DISCHARGE DIAGNOSIS: Asthma with exacerbation

DISCHARGE INSTRUCTIONS: The patient was instructed to take his prescribed medications as directed by his primary care physician and to return to the ER if he had any further asthma.

PATIENT 8

ICD-9-CM CODES

PDX					.		
DX2					.		
DX3					.		
DX4					.		

CPT CODES

PP1					
PR2					
PR3					
PR4					
PR5					
PR6					
PR7					

OTHER AMBULATORY RECORDS—Patients 9 A and B

Patient 9 A

Right and Left Heart Catheterization and Coronary Angiography

PROCEDURE: After obtaining informed consent the patient was taken to the cardiac catheterization laboratory. The right groin was prepped and draped in the usual fashion and 2% Xylocaine was used to anesthetize. 6-French sheaths were introduced into the right femoral artery and vein and a 6-French multipurpose catheter was used for the heart catheterization, coronary angiography, and ventricular angiography. Right heart pressures and cardiac outputs were measured. A pigtail catheter was inserted into the left ventricular cavity and ventricular pressures obtained. Angiography of the right coronary artery was performed. Left ventricular angiography and aortic root angiography was performed. The patient tolerated the procedure well without complications.

DIAGNOSIS: Arteriosclerotic coronary artery disease

PATIENT 9 A

ICD-9-CM CODES

PDX							
DX2							
DX3							
DX4							

CPT CODES

PP1					
PR2					
PR3					
PR4					
PR5					
PR6					
PR7					

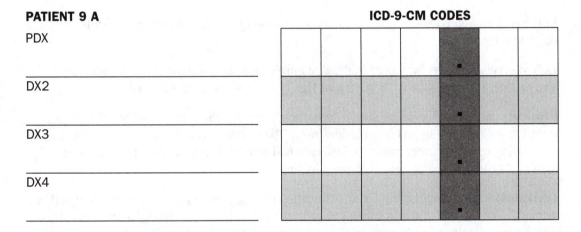

Patient 9 B

Left Heart Catherization, Left Ventriculography, Coronary Angiography, Drug-Eluting Stent to Left Anterior Descending Coronary Artery

PROCEDURE: After obtaining informed consent the patient was taken to the cardiac catherizations laboratory. He was prepped and draped in the usual fashion and 2% Xylocaine was used to anesthetize the right groin. 6-French sheaths were introduced into the right femoral artery and vein and a 6-French multipurpose catheter was used for left heart catheterizations, coronary angiography, and left ventricular angiography. I then proceeded to perform a Stent/PTCA to the LAD. A HTF wire was used to cross the LAD stenosis and a 4.0-mm J&J stent was placed in the left anterior descending coronary vessel with excellent results. The final angiogram was obtained and the guiding catheterization was removed. The sheaths were securely sutured and the patient tolerated the procedure well without complications.

FINDINGS:

Left heart catheterizations revealed an elevated resting left ventricular end diastolic pressure of 18 mm Hg.

Left ventriculography is viewed in the RAO projection with normal systolic wall motion. The end-diastolic pressure is 18 to 20 mm Hg. There is no gradient detected.

Coronary angiography (using single catheter): The right coronary vessel has dominant structure with minor luminal irregularities only. The left main is normal with the left anterior descending coronary artery having a 75% calcified proximal stenosis and the circumflex marginal system with a 10% to 20% plaquing only.

LAD stent underlying: Left anterior descending coronary vessel was easily isolated and the primary stent intervention was carried out with a 3.0 Cypher drug-eluting stent. Final sizing was 3.1 mm resulting in 0% residual stenosis and maintenance of TIMI III flow distally in the LAD system.

IMPRESSION: Critical single-vessel obstructive coronary artery disease involving the LAD system successfully treated with drug-eluting stent technology. The left anterior descending coronary artery shows excellent results. Preserved left ventricular systolic wall motion.

PATIENT 9 B

ICD-9-CM CODES

PDX					.		
DX2					.		
DX3					.		
DX4					.		

CPT CODES

PP1					
PR2					
PR3					
PR4					
PR5					
PR6					
PR7					

OTHER AMBULATORY RECORDS—Patients 10 A and B

INTERVENTIONAL RADIOLOGY REPORT—Patient 10 A

EXAMINATION: US Guided Liver Biopsy

HISTORY: Carcinoma of the lung

PROCEDURE: Limited real-time transabdominal ultrasound of the liver was performed. There is a 3.5 × 2.9-cm mass in the lateral segment of the left lobe of the liver. This mass is hypoechogenic with increased blood flow. Following informed consent the patient was prepped and draped in the usual manner. Using ultrasound guidance, percutaneous fine-needle aspiration biopsy of the left lobe of the liver mass was performed. The patient tolerated the procedure well.

IMPRESSION: Hypoechogenic mass in the left lobe of the liver that was successfully biopsied with ultrasound guidance.

PATHOLOGY REPORT: Consistent with metastatic lung carcinoma

PATIENT 10 A

ICD-9-CM CODES

PDX

DX2

DX3

DX4

CPT CODES

PP1

PR2

PR3

PR4

PR5

PR6

PR7

PAIN MANAGEMENT—EPIDURAL STEROID INJECTION—Patient 10 B

DIAGNOSIS: Low back pain, lumbar radiculopathy with chronic pain syndrome

HISTORY: This is an 18-year-old white female with low back pain and lumbar radicular pain for epidural steroid injection. The patient had an epidural approximately three weeks ago with approximately 30% improvement. The patient is agreeable for additional epidural steroid injection for pain management.

PROCEDURE: Epidural steroid injection under C-arm guidance via caudal approach and epidurogram. The patient was transferred to the operating room and placed in the prone position. Under MAC anesthesia her low back and sacral areas were sterilely prepped and draped. Local 1% lidocaine was applied with a #23-gauge needle through the skin and surrounding tissues of the sacral hiatus. Then a #17-gauge Epimed needle was inserted percutaneously through the sacral hiatus into the epidural space. This was confirmed via lateral view of the C-arm. Then under AP fluoroscopy, an #18-gauge Epimed catheter was guided to the mid L3-L4 area of the nerve root in the midline. Next, 2 cc of Isovue dye was injected, which showed good bilateral spread in the epidural space. A solution of 6 cc of normal saline, 80 mg of Depo-Medrol and 2 cc of 1% lidocaine was partially deposited at the L3-L4 nerve root. The catheter was then moved down to the L4-L5 nerve root in the midline of the epidural space. An additional 1 cc of Isovue dye was injected, which showed good bilateral spread. An additional one third of local anesthetic Depo-Medrol solution was deposited at the L4-L5 nerve root. The catheter was then moved down to the L5-S1 nerve root and in the midline. Another 1 cc of Isovue dye was injected, which confirmed good bilateral spread and highlighting of the L5-S1 nerve roots bilateral. The remaining local anesthetic Depo-Medrol solution was deposited at the L5-S1 nerve root. The catheter and needle were then pulled intact and the patient was transferred to the recovery room in satisfactory condition.

IMPRESSION: Low back pain, lumbar radiculopathy. This is the patient's second epidural steroid injection.

FOLLOW-UP: After seeing improvement in the next 24 to 48 hours and repeat injection if necessary.

PATIENT 10 B

ICD-9-CM CODES

PDX					.		
DX2					.		
DX3					.		
DX4					.		

CPT CODES

PP1					
PR2					
PR3					
PR4					
PR5					
PR6					
PR7					

OTHER AMBULATORY RECORD—Patient 11 A

DATE: 8/12/200X

SURGERY RECORD:

PATIENT HISTORY: This patient is seen today to insert an intrathecal pump for pain management due to ductal carcinoma of the left upper lobe of the breast metastatic to the spine. She underwent modified radical mastectomy with general anesthesia and had no adverse effects. No other surgical history is given. No known allergies, no current medications. Review of systems is normal ASA = 2.

Following preoperative evaluation and discussion with the patient, local anesthesia was used to implant an intrathecal programmable pump. The patient tolerated the procedure well. There were no adverse effects of anesthesia.

Please code the diagnosis and CPT code(s).

PATIENT 11 A

ICD-9-CM CODES

PDX					.		
DX2					.		
DX3					.		
DX4					.		

CPT CODES

PP1					
PR2					
PR3					
PR4					
PR5					
PR6					
PR7					

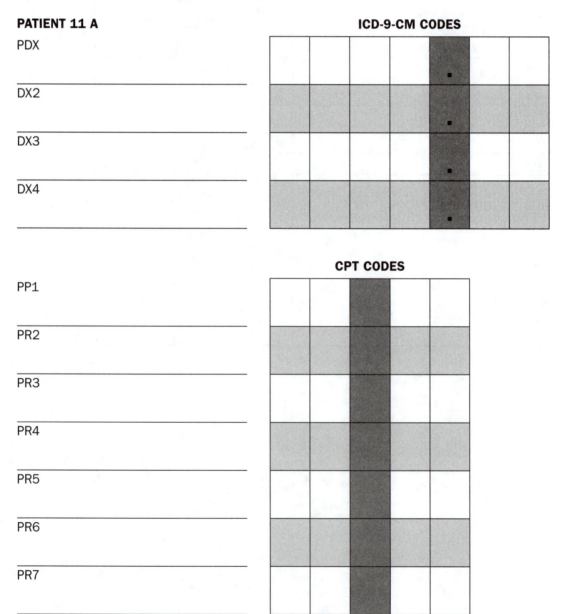

OTHER AMBULATORY RECORD—Patient 11 B

PREOPERATIVE DIAGNOSIS: Reflex sympathetic dystrophy, left knee

POSTOPERATIVE DIAGNOSIS: Reflex sympathetic dystrophy, left knee

OPERATION: Left lumbar sympathetic block with C-arm

ANESTHESIA: Local

INDICATIONS:

This 43-year-old female has a seven-month history of left knee pain. She says that even light touch appears to be exquisitely painful. She has had surgery to clear scar tissue.

PROCEDURE DESCRIPTION:

The patient was placed on the x-ray lucent gurney in the right lateral decubitus position. The back was prepped with Betadine, and the midline spinous processes were marked. A line was drawn 6 to 7 cm lateral to that midline on the left. L2 was identified using the C-arm and lateral projections, and lidocaine was infiltrated at the skin. The 22-gauge, 6-inch Chiba needle was advanced down to and off the body of L2, and loss of resistance was obtained with a glass syringe. Renografin-60 was injected and showed a good distribution. So 15 cc of bupivacaine 0.5% without epinephrine was injected, plus Depo-Medrol 40 mg. The needle was withdrawn.

Then lidocaine was infiltrated on the 6 to 7-cm line at L4. I advanced the 22-gauge, 6-inch needle off the body of L4, but the Renografin-60 distribution appeared not to be adequate. Another wheal was raised at the 13 level, and the needle was advanced down to and off the body of L3. A loss of resistance was obtained with a glass syringe, followed by Renografin-60. This time, the distribution was excellent, and bupivacaine 0.5% without epinephrine × 15 cc was injected. She was left on her side for 25 minutes. After 10 minutes, she had a noticeably warmer left foot and ankle. The skin coloration of the left leg was normal.

Please code the diagnosis and CPT code(s).

PATIENT 11 B

PDX

DX2

DX3

DX4

ICD-9-CM CODES

				.		
				.		
				.		
				.		

PP1

PR2

PR3

PR4

PR5

PR6

PR7

CPT CODES

Part II: Inpatient Cases

If you need practice coding delivery records, skip records 12 and 13 and code 12 A and 13 A.

Instructions and official coding guidelines for coding medical records are included in the following resources:

- ICD-9-CM codebook coding conventions, alphabetical, and tabular indices
- *ICD-9-CM Official Guidelines* for coding and reporting
- *Coding Clinic for ICD-9-CM* (AHA)
- *Coding Clinic for HCPCS* (AHA)
- Additional coding guidance can be found in the *CPT Assistant* (AMA)

Hospitals and other organizations may develop their own procedures in the absence of approved guidelines. To ensure consistent coding, the following procedures have been developed for use in the CCS exam. The procedures do not supersede or replace official coding advice and guidelines included in the resources identified above.

These procedures are to be used only in completing the CCS examination. They will be provided to candidates as part of the examination packet. Not adhering to these procedures may result in the miscoding of an exercise, which may result in the deduction of points when the item is scored.

Inpatient Coding Procedures

1. Apply UHDDS definitions, ICD-9-CM instructional notations and conventions, and current approved national ICD-9-CM coding guidelines to assign correct ICD-9-CM diagnostic and procedural codes to hospital inpatient medical records.
2. Sequence the ICD-9-CM codes, listing the principal diagnosis first.
3. Code other diagnoses that coexist at the time of admission, that develop subsequently, or that affect the treatment received and/or the length of stay. These represent additional conditions that affect patient care in terms of requiring clinical evaluation, therapeutic treatment, diagnostic procedures, extended length of hospital stay, or increased nursing care and/or monitoring.
   A. Code diagnoses that require active intervention during hospitalization. For example: Admission for small-bowel ileus and subsequent aspiration pneumonia that is treated with antibiotics and respiratory therapy. Code the ileus and aspiration pneumonia.
   B. Code diagnoses that require active management of chronic disease during hospitalization, which is defined as a patient who continues on chronic management at time of hospitalization. For example: Admission for acute exacerbation of COPD. The patient has depression that extends the stay and for which psychiatric consultation is obtained. Code the COPD and depression. For example: Admission for acute exacerbation of COPD. Physician lists "history of depression" on the face sheet, and the patient is given Desyrel. Code the COPD and depression.
   C. Code diagnoses of chronic systemic or generalized conditions that are not under active management when a physician documents them in the record and that may have a bearing on the management of the patient. For example: Admission for

breast mass; diagnosis is carcinoma. Patient is blind and requires increased care. Code the breast carcinoma and blindness.

D. Code status post previous surgeries or conditions likely to recur that may have a bearing on the management of the patient. For example: Admission for pneumonia; status post cardiac bypass surgery. Code the pneumonia and status post cardiac bypass surgery (V code).

E. Do not code status post previous surgeries or histories of conditions that have no bearing on the management of the patient. For example: Admission for pneumonia; status post hernia repair six months prior to admission. Code only the pneumonia.

F. Do not code localized conditions that have no bearing on the management of the patient. For example: Admission for hernia repair; the patient has a nevus on his leg that is not treated or evaluated. Code only the hernia and its repair.

G. Do not code abnormal findings (laboratory, x-ray, pathologic, and other diagnostic results) unless there is documentary evidence from the physician of their clinical significance. For example: Admission for elective joint replacement for degenerative joint disease. The laboratory report shows a serum sodium of 133; no further documentation addresses this laboratory result. Code only the degenerative joint disease and the replacement surgery. For example: Admission for elective joint replacement for degenerative joint disease. The laboratory report shows a low potassium level, and the physician documents hypokalemia. Intravenous potassium was administered by the physician for hypokalemia. Code the degenerative joint disease, the replacement surgery, and hypokalemia.

H. Do not code symptoms and signs that are characteristic of a diagnosis. For example: A patient has dyspnea due to COPD. Code only the COPD.

I. Do not code condition(s) in the Social History section that has no bearing on the management of the patient.

4. Do not assign External Cause of Injury and Poisoning Codes (E codes), except those that identify the causative substance for an adverse effect of a drug that is correctly prescribed and properly administered (E930–E949).
5. Do not assign Morphology codes (M codes).
6. Code all procedures that fall within the code range 01.01–86.99, but do not code 57.94 (Foley catheter).
7. Do not code procedures that fall within the code range 87.01–99.99. But code procedures in the following ranges:

87.51–87.54	Cholangiograms
87.74 and 87.76	Retrogrades, urinary systems
88.40–88.58	Arteriography and angiography
92.21–92.29	Radiation therapy
94.24–94.27	Psychiatric therapy
94.61–94.69	Alcohol/drug detoxification and rehabilitation
96.04	Insertion of endotracheal tube
96.70–96.72	Mechanical ventilation
98.51–98.59	ESWL
99.25	Chemotherapy

INPATIENT RECORD—Patient 12

DISCHARGE SUMMARY

DATE OF ADMISSION: 11/30 **DATE OF DISCHARGE**: 12/4

DISCHARGE DIAGNOSIS: Fractured neck of right femur

ADMISSION HISTORY: The patient is a 78-year-old male who fell on the day of admission and sustained a fracture of the neck of his right femur. The patient was admitted for a medical evaluation prior to surgical intervention.

COURSE IN HOSPITAL: Medical evaluation was obtained on admission. Patient was taken to the operating room, where an open reduction and internal fixation of the fracture of the right femur was performed. Postoperative course was unremarkable except for urinary retention, which necessitated the placement of an indwelling Foley catheter. He was discharged with the catheter in place. The patient was ambulatory, non-weight bearing with a walker at the time of discharge.

INSTRUCTIONS ON DISCHARGE: The patient is instructed to follow-up with my office in 3 days to remove staples and to begin outpatient physical therapy tomorrow. Home health services will follow this patient. Pain medications: Darvocet N 100, one tablet every 4 hours as needed for pain.

HISTORY AND PHYSICAL EXAMINATION—Patient 12

ADMITTED: 11/30

REASON FOR ADMISSION: Right hip pain following a fall

HISTORY OF PRESENT ILLNESS: The patient is a 78-year-old male who fell on the day of admission and sustained a fracture of the neck of his right femur. The patient was admitted for a medical evaluation prior to surgical intervention.

PAST MEDICAL HISTORY: The patient has had multiple medical problems including gastric ulcer, congestive heart failure, diverticulosis, degenerative joint disease, arteriosclerotic coronary artery disease, and mitral regurgitation.

ALLERGIES: None

CHRONIC MEDICATIONS: Lanoxin .125 mg, Mon. Wed., and Fri., Lasix 40 mg q. a.m., Lasix 40 mg q. p.m., Colace 200 mg q. a.m., Metamucil one teaspoon b.i.d., Zestril 10 mg every day, Zantac 150 mg PO b.i.d., nitroglycerin 0.4 mg. PRN for chest pain, Celebrex 100 mg PO b.i.d. for degenerative joint disease.

SOCIAL HISTORY: The patient is widowed with 3 children and 7 grandchildren. The patient is a nondrinker and nonsmoker.

REVIEW OF SYSTEMS: The patient has been in usual health until the day prior to admission when he fell. There has been no change in bladder and bowel functioning. Cognitively, he has experienced some confusion on and off lately.

PHYSICAL EXAMINATION: BP is 170/90, pulse 80 and regular. The patient is an elderly, thin, somewhat deaf male. His pupils are small and reactive to light. The pharynx is benign. The jugular pulse is distended but filled from above. He has no supraclavicular adenopathy. His chest is clear. On palpation the pericardium was located in his anterior axillary line with a palpable thrill. On auscultation he had a harsh grade III/VI apical systolic murmur that radiated to the apex and faintly to the lower left sternal edge. He had a soft diastolic flow murmur. His abdomen was somewhat tense without organomegaly. He had minimal peripheral edema.

CONSULTATION—Patient 12

DATE: 11/30

CHIEF COMPLAINT: Pain in hip

REVIEW OF SYSTEMS: The patient has been in usual health until the day prior to admission when he fell. The patient is experiencing a little more shortness of breath than usual. The patient is unsure if he felt dizzy before falling.

PHYSICAL EXAMINATION: This is an elderly, moderately nourished white male. HEENT reveals nothing abnormal. There is no adenopathy. His chest is clear with loud grade III/VI pansystolic murmur. Examination of the abdomen reveals no masses or tenderness. He had minimal peripheral edema with one leg appearing shorter than the other. Distal circulation and sensation are normal.

IMPRESSION:

History of gastric ulcer
Congestive heart failure
Diverticulosis
Degenerative joint disease
Arteriosclerotic coronary artery disease
Mitral regurgitation

PLAN: D/C NSAIDs for now in light of GI history. The patient is cleared for surgery.

PROGRESS NOTES—Patient 12

DATE	NOTE
11/30	Patient admitted for medical evaluation prior to ORIF. The patient is somewhat confused about the events surrounding the fall. At present he offers no other complaint. The patient currently has Bucks traction in place. If cleared for surgery, patient is scheduled for tomorrow at 1:00 p.m.
12/1	The patient is resting quietly. Medication adequate to alleviate pain in extremity.
6:30 a.m.	Operative consent signed following obtaining informed consent for surgery. All questions from patient and family answered.
	PREOP DX: Fracture of right femur
6:30 p.m.	POSTOP DX: Same
	OPERATION: Open reduction, internal fixation, fracture, right hip
	ANESTHESIA: Spinal and general
	COMPLICATIONS: None
	Patient sleeping. Dressings intact, hemovac in place.
8:00 p.m.	House Physician called to see patient due to inability to void. The patient appears to have postop urinary retention. Will place Foley catheter.
10:00 p.m.	
12/2	Events of last night noted. Will request that patient get OOB and begin physical therapy. Hemovac in place draining small amount. Patient not complaining of pain. H&H looks good. Lytes fine.
12/3	Patient has been ambulating well. Patient minimally confused due to senile dementia. Neurovascular status good. Appetite good. Dressing intact, incision healing well, no redness or inflammation.
12/4	Patient up with assistance and ambulating using walker. Incision healing well. Discharge with indwelling Foley. Home health services to assist patient following discharge. Ready for discharge today.

PHYSICIAN'S ORDERS—Patient 12

DATE	ORDER

11/30	Admit to floor
	NPO after midnight
	Continue present meds:
	    Lanoxin 0.125 mg, q.d
	    Lasix 40 mg q. a.m. and p.m.
	    Colace 200 mg q. a.m.
	    Metamucil one teaspoon b.i.d.
	    Zantac 150 mg po b.i.d.
	    Celebrex 100 mg po b.i.d. for DJD
	Prep for hip surgery
	Medical Consult for surgical clearance
	4 lb Bucks traction to continue
	Demerol 50 mg q. 3 to 4 hours
	Darvocet N 100 q. 3 to 4 hours
	Cross match 3 units of blood
	Low sodium, low-fat diet
	Dig level in a.m.
	H&H and electrolytes

12/1	Preop Meds
	Hold Dig this a.m.
	Ancef 1 g on call to OR
	Postop Meds
	    Run D5W 1,000 cc q. 12 hrs
	    Demerol 500 mg q. 3 to 4 hrs p.r.n. pain
	    Darvocet N 100 q. 3 to 4 hours
	    Hct and Hgb at 9:00 p.m. and in a.m.
	    Electrolytes in a.m.
	    Ancef 500 mg IV q. 6 hrs × 4 doses
	X-ray hip in a.m.
	Ice on hip
	Up in chair following x-ray
	Begin physical therapy tomorrow
	Insert Foley catheter

12/2	Consult home health services for discharge needs. Continue pain meds. Get patient OOB for ambulation with walker.
12/3	D/C IV
12/4	D/C patient. Home health services to follow.

OPERATIVE REPORT—Patient 12

DATE: 12/1

PREOPERATIVE DIAGNOSIS: Fracture of right femur

POSTOPERATIVE DIAGNOSIS: Same

OPERATION: Open reduction and internal fixation of fracture right hip

ANESTHESIA: Spinal and general

OPERATIVE INDICATIONS:

OPERATIVE PROCEDURE: The patient was given Ancef 1 g IV 30 minutes prior to the procedure for endocarditis/surgical prophylaxis. The patient was administered a spinal anesthesia and then placed on the fracture table in traction. X-rays revealed satisfactory position and alignment of the fracture site. The right hip was prepped with Betadine scrub and Betadine solution and draped in a sterile fashion. A straight incision was made over the lateral aspect of the right hip and carried through the subcutaneous tissue, then tensor fascia lata and vastus lateralis muscles so that the fracture could be reduced and fixation devices utilized. The lateral shaft of the femur was exposed subperiosteally. A guide wire was then placed into the neck and head of the femur and x-rays revealed a slightly inferior position. The new guide wire was obtained in satisfactory position. The lateral shaft, neck, and head of the femur were then drilled to a depth of 85 mm with the drill. An 85-mm, 140-degree and 5-degree compression nail were then inserted over which a 140-degree angle 4 hole side plate was then inserted. A compression screw was then applied after the key was inserted. The side plate was then fixed to the shaft of the femur with four screws. X-rays revealed satisfactory position and alignment of the fracture fragments and the fixation device. The wound was then well irrigated. A large hemovac drain was inserted and brought out through a separate stab wound incision. The wound was closed with a continuous #000 Vicryl suture in the vastus lateralis and tensor fascia lata layers. The subcutaneous tissue was closed with interrupted #000 Vicryl sutures and the skin was closed with staples. A compression dressing was applied. The patient tolerated the procedure well and there were no operative complications. Patient was returned to the recovery room in satisfactory condition.

LABORATORY REPORTS—Patient 12

HEMATOLOGY

DATE: 11/30

Specimen	Results	Normal Values
WBC	09.9	4.3–11.0
RBC	5.0	4.5–5.9
HGB	14.0	13.5–17.5
HCT	45	41–52
MCV	89	80–100
MCHC	33.9	31–57
PLT	Adequate	

HEMATOLOGY

DATE: 12/1

Specimen	Results	Normal Values
WBC	7.7	4.3–11.0
RBC	4.4 L	4.5–5.9
HGB	13.2 L	13.5–17.5
HCT	41	41–52
MCV	89	80–100
MCHC	33.9	31–57
PLT	Adequate	

HEMATOLOGY

DATE: 12/1

Specimen	Results	Normal Values
WBC	08.0	4.3–11.0
RBC	4.5	4.5–5.9
HGB	13.7	13.5–17.5
HCT	42	41–52
MCV	89	80–100
MCHC	33.9	31–57
PLT	Adequate	

LABORATORY REPORT—Patient 12

CHEMISTRY

DATE: 11/30

Specimen	Results	Normal Values
GLUC	97	70–110
BUN	12	8–25
CREAT	1.0	0.5–1.5
NA	138	136-146
K	4.0	3.5–5.5
CL	109	95–110
CO2	33 H	24–32
CA	9.1	8.4–10.5
PHOS	3.0	2.5–4.4
MG	2.0	1.6–3.0
T BILI	1.0	0.2–1.2
D BILI	0.4	0.0–0.5
PROTEIN	7.0	6.0–8.0
ALBUMIN	5.4	5.0–5.5
AST	36	0–40
ALT	44	30–65
GCT	70	15–85
LD	110	100–190
ALK PHOS	114	50–136
URIC ACID	6.0	2.2–7.7
CHOL	165	0–200
TRIG	140	10–160

CHEMISTRY

DATE: 12/1

Specimen	Results	Normal Values
GLUC	97	70–110
BUN	12	8–25
CREAT	1.0	0.5–1.5
NA	134 L	136–146
K	5.6 H	3.5–5.5
CL	109	95–110
CO2	33 H	24–32
CA	9.1	8.4–10.5
PHOS	3.0	2.5–4.4
MG	2.0	1.6–3.0
T BILI	1.0	0.2–1.2
D BILI	0.4	0.0–0.5
PROTEIN	7.0	6.0–8.0
ALBUMIN	5.4	5.0–5.5
AST	36	0–40
ALT	44	30–65
GGT	70	15–85
LD	110	100–190
ALK PHOS	114	50–136
URIC ACID	6.0	2.2–7.7
CHOL	165	0–200
TRIG	140	10–160

RADIOLOGY REPORT—Patient 12

DATE: 11/30

RIGHT HIP AND FEMUR: A displaced intertrochanteric fracture is noted with a mild degree of varus angulation. The adjacent skeletal structures are normal. The right femur is intact beyond the hip. There is vascular calcification.

CHEST, SUPINE: There is no gross evidence of acute inflammatory disease or congestive heart failure.

IMPRESSION: Femur and hip; slightly angulated intertrochanteric fracture Chest; no acute disease

RADIOLOGY REPORT—Patient 12

DATE: 12/2

DIAGNOSIS: RIGHT HIP AND FEMUR: The displaced intertrochanteric fracture has been surgically corrected. The adjacent skeletal structures are normal.

IMPRESSION: The fracture is maintained with an orthopedic device.

PATIENT 12

ICD-9-CM CODES

PDX					.		
DX2					.		
DX3					.		
DX4					.		
DX5					.		
DX6					.		
DX7					.		
DX8					.		
DX9					.		
DX10					.		

ICD-9-CM CODES

PP1			.		
PR2			.		
PR3			.		
PR4			.		
PR5			.		
PR6			.		

INPATIENT RECORD

DISCHARGE SUMMARY—Patient 12 A

DATE OF ADMISSION: 2/3 **DATE OF DISCHARGE**: 2/5

DISCHARGE DIAGNOSIS: Full-term pregnancy—delivered male infant

Patient started labor spontaneously three days before her due date. She was brought to the hospital by automobile. Labor progressed for a while but then contractions became fewer and she delivered soon after. A midline episiotomy was done. Membranes and placenta were complete. There was some bleeding but not excessive. Patient made an uneventful recovery.

HISTORY AND PHYSICAL EXAMINATION—Patient 12 A

ADMITTED: 2/3

REASON FOR ADMISSION: Full-term pregnancy

PAST MEDICAL HISTORY: Previous deliveries normal and mitral valve prolapse

ALLERGIES: None known

CHRONIC MEDICATIONS: None

FAMILY HISTORY: Heart disease—Father

SOCIAL HISTORY: The patient is married and has one other child living with her.

REVIEW OF SYSTEMS:

SKIN: Normal

HEAD-SCALP: Normal

EYES: Normal

ENT: Normal

NECK: Normal

BREASTS: Normal

THORAX: Normal

LUNGS: Normal

HEART: Slight midsystolic click with late systolic murmur II/VI

ABDOMEN: Normal

IMPRESSION: Good health with term pregnancy. History of mitral valve prolapse—asymptomatic

PROGRESS NOTES—Patient 12 A

DATE	NOTE
2/3	Admit to Labor and Delivery. MVP stable. Patient progressing well. Delivered at 1:15 p.m. one full-term male infant.
2/4	Patient doing well. MVP prolapse stable. The perineum is clean and dry, incision intact.
2/5	Will discharge to home

PHYSICIAN'S ORDERS—Patient 12 A

DATE	ORDER
2/3	Admit to Labor and Delivery 1,000 cc 5% D/LR May ambulate Type and screen CBC May have ice chips
2/5	Discharge patient to home

DELIVERY RECORD—Patient 12 A

DATE: 2/3

The patient was 3 cm dilated when admitted. The duration of the first stage of labor was 6 hours, second stage was 14 minutes, third stage was 5 minutes. She was given local anesthesia. An episiotomy was performed with repair. There were no lacerations. The cord was wrapped once around the baby's neck, but did not cause compression. The mother and liveborn baby were discharged from the delivery room in good condition.

LABORATORY REPORT—Patient 12 A

HEMATOLOGY

DATE: 2/3

Specimen	Results	Normal Values
WBC	5.2	4.3–11.0
RBC	4.9	4.5–5.9
HGB	13.8	13.5–17.5
HCT	45	41–52
MCV	93	80–100
MCHC	41	31–57
PLT	255	150–400

PATIENT 12 A

ICD-9-CM CODES

PDX					.		
DX2					.		
DX3					.		
DX4					.		
DX5					.		
DX6					.		
DX7					.		
DX8					.		
DX9					.		
DX10					.		

ICD-9-CM CODES

PP1			.		
PR2			.		
PR3			.		
PR4			.		
PR5			.		
PR6			.		

INPATIENT RECORD

DISCHARGE SUMMARY—Patient 13

DATE OF ADMISSION: 1/31 **DATE OF DISCHARGE**: 2/3

DISCHARGE DIAGNOSIS: Right lower lobe pneumonia due to gram-negative bacteria, resistant to erythromycin

ADMISSION HISTORY: This is a 56-year-old insulin-requiring diabetic female whom we have been following for hypertension, degenerative joint disease, aortic stenosis and diabetic retinopathy. Over the past three days she has noted increased cough and chest congestion with a fever of approximately 102 degrees. She was found to have a right lower lobe infiltrate and was started on therapy with erythromycin. Despite initial therapy, the patient's clinical status has worsened over the past 24 hours.

COURSE IN HOSPITAL: Patient was admitted with the diagnosis of right lower lobe pneumonia. She was begun on intravenous ceftriaxone. Because of difficulties with venous access, patient was switched to intramuscular ceftriaxone on her third hospital day.

By 2/3 the patient was afebrile and her cough had diminished. Her blood pressure was well controlled at 140/74.

INSTRUCTIONS ON DISCHARGE: Follow-up with me by phone in three days and in my office in two weeks. Repeat chest x-ray to be done then.

MEDICATIONS:
1. Calan SR 180 mg b.i.d.;
2. Zestril 20 mg PO q. a.m.;
3. NPH Insulin, 30 units, sub q., a.m.;
4. Levoquin 500 mg PO daily × 10 days.;
5. Celebrex 100 mg PO b.i.d.

HISTORY AND PHYSICAL EXAMINATION—Patient 13

ADMITTED: 1/31

REASON FOR ADMISSION: Physical examination on admission revealed a well-developed, acutely ill appearing black female.

HISTORY OF PRESENT ILLNESS: A 56-year-old diabetic followed for hypertension and diabetic retinopathy. Over the past three days she has noted increased cough and chest congestion with a fever of approximately 102 degrees. She was found to have a right lower lobe infiltrate and was begun on therapy with erythromycin. Despite initial therapy, the patient's clinical status worsened over the past 24 hours and hospitalization was recommended.

PAST MEDICAL HISTORY: Hypertension, degenerative joint disease in both knees, and moderate aortic stenosis.

ALLERGIES: Dust

CHRONIC MEDICATIONS: CalanSR 180 mg po b.i.d., Insulin (NPH), Zestril 20 mg PO daily, Celebrex 100 mg PO b.i.d.

FAMILY HISTORY: Notable for hypertension in mother

SOCIAL HISTORY: Noncontributory

PHYSICAL EXAMINATION:

GENERAL APPEARANCE: The patient is a well-developed black female in moderate distress.

VITAL SIGNS: T 102, P 80, R 16, BP 150/80

SKIN: Warm and dry

HEENT: Significant for mildly inflamed mucous membranes. Retinopathy evident in both eyes.

NECK: Supple. Symmetrical with no bruits

LUNGS: Coarse rhonchi bilaterally, right greater than left

HEART: Regular rate and rhythm, positive S1, positive III/VI SEM

ABDOMEN: Soft, nontender, no mass

GENITALIA: Deferred

RECTAL: Deferred

EXTREMITIES: No edema

NEUROLOGIC: Normal

HISTORY AND PHYSICAL EXAMINATION—Patient 13

LABORATORY DATA:

1. EKG: NSR, widespread ST-T wave abnormalities, LV hypertrophy
2. CBC: Hgb 13, Hct 38, WBC 12.8
3. Glucose: 281
4. Urinalysis: Unremarkable
5. Sputum: Gram stain—a few WBCs, moderate gram-negative rods

IMPRESSION:

1. Right Lower Lobe Pneumonia possibly due to gram-negative bacteria
2. Diabetes Mellitus on Insulin—Uncontrolled
3. Hypertension—Stable
4. Degenerative Joint Disease—Stable
5. Moderate Aortic Stenosis

PLAN: Admit, IV antibiotics for pneumonia. Monitor blood sugars

PROGRESS NOTES—Patient 13

DATE	NOTE
1/31	Patient admitted for cough associated with increased temperature with chest x-ray indicative of pneumonia. Will obtain sputum culture and begin on ceftriaxone. Will monitor blood pressure and blood sugars. Will use sliding scale to bring blood sugar into control. Patient with recent echocardiogram as outpatient that showed stable aortic stenosis.
2/1	The patient is responding well. Will request diabetic education nurse to meet with her and set up an appointment for classes following this admission.
2/2	Sputum culture reveals gram-negative bacteria as suspected. Patient's temperature is down. Patient resting comfortably. Blood sugar better.
2/3	Blood sugar with increasing control today. The importance of appropriate diet emphasized. Will discharge with p.o. antibiotics.

PHYSICIAN'S ORDERS—Patient 13

DATE	ORDER
1/31/200X	Admit to 3 South DX: Pneumonia Please give ceftriaxone 1 g q 8 hours IV ADA diet CBC and SMA CalanSR 50 mg in a.m. with orange juice Zestril 2 in a.m. Celebrex 100 mg po BID Accucheck before meals and before bedtime Chest x-ray Sliding scale for insulin as follows: below 120 give 4 units of regular 120–200 give 6 units of Regular insulin 200–300 give 8 units of Regular insulin Above 300 call physician
2/1/9x	Change insulin to 40 NPH units sq in a.m. today Consult diabetic nurse to see patient and set up classes following admission
2/2/9x	Continue insulin to 40 NPH units sq in a.m. today
2/2/9x	D/C IV and switch to ceftriaxone 1 g IM q. 24 hrs
2/3/9x	Discharge to home.

LABORATORY REPORTS—Patient 13

MICROBIOLOGY

DATE	TEST TYPE	
1/31/200X	SOURCE:	
	SITE:	
	GRAM STAIN RESULTS: Sputum	
	CULTURE RESULTS: Slight WBC's, Slight Epi's	
	Many gram-negative rods	
	sl. gram-negative diplococci	
	sl. gram-positive cocci in clusters	
DATE	SUSCEPTIBILITY:	S
	AMPICILLIN	S
	CEFAZOLIN	S
	CEFOTAXIME	S
	CEFTRIAXONE	S
	CEFUROXIME	S
	CEPHALOTHIN	S
	CIPROFLOXACIN	S
	ERYTHROMYCIN	R
	GENTAMICIN	S
	OXACILLIN	S
	PENICILLIN	S
	PIPERACILLIN	S
	TETRACYCLINE	S
	TOBRAMYCIN	S
	TRIMETH/SULF	S
	VANCOMYCIN	S

S = SUSCEPTIBLE
R = RESISTANT
I = INTERMEDIATE
M = MODERATELY SUSCEP

RADIOLOGY REPORT—Patient 13

DATE: 1/31/200X

HISTORY DIAGNOSIS: Pneumonia

FINDINGS: There is slight overexpansion of the lungs. The pulmonary vasculature is normal. The heart is not enlarged. There is lower lobe infiltrate in the right lung.

IMPRESSION: Right lower lobe pneumonia

EKG REPORT—Patient 13

DATE: 1/31/200X

DIAGNOSIS: Pneumonia

INTERPRETATION:

EKG: NSR, widespread ST-T wave abnormalities, LV hypertrophy

LABORATORY REPORT—Patient 13

CHEMISTRY

DATE: 1/31/200X

Specimen	Results	Normal Values
GLUC	281 H	70–110
CREAT	0.67	0.5–1.5
NA	142	136–146
K	4.8	3.5–5.5
CL	108	95–110
CO2	29	24–32
CA	9.5	8.4–10.5
PHOS	3.8	2.5–4.4
MG	2.8	1.6–3.0
T BILI	1.0	0.2–1.2
D BILI	0.3	0.0–0.5
PROTEIN	6.5	6.0–8.0
ALBUMIN	5.1	5.0–5.5
AST	38	0–40
ALT	54	30–65
GGT	50	15–85
LD	180	100–190
ALK PHOS	102	50–136
URIC ACID	4.5	2.2–7.7
CHOL	89	0–200
TRIG	101	10–160

LABORATORY REPORT—Patient 13

URINALYSIS

DATE: 1/31

Test	Result	Ref Range
SP GRAVITY	1.007	1.005–1.035
PH	7.0	5–7
PROT	NEG	NEG
GLUC	NEG	NEG
KETONES	NEG	NEG
BILI	NEG	NEG
BLOOD	NEG	NEG
LEU EST	NEG	NEG
NITRATES	NEG	NEG
RED SUBS	NEG	NEG

LABORATORY REPORTS—Patient 13

HEMATOLOGY

DATE: 1/31

Specimen	Results	Normal Values
WBC	12.8 H	4.3–11.0
RBC	5.5	4.5–5.9
HGB	13.0 L	13.5–17.5
HCT	38 L	41–52
MCV	90	80–100
MCHC	41	31–57
PLT	251	150–400

BLOOD GLUCOSE MONITORING RECORD—Patient 13

1/31	11:00 a.m.	310
	4:00 p.m.	300
	9:00 p.m.	290
2/1	7:00 a.m.	150
	11:00 a.m.	175
	4:00 p.m.	145
	9:00 p.m.	175
2/2	7:00 a.m.	140
	11:00 a.m.	135
	4:00 p.m.	160
	9:00 p.m.	150
2/3	7:00 a.m.	135
	11:00 a.m.	150
	4:00 p.m.	130

PATIENT 13

ICD-9-CM CODES

PDX					.		
DX2					.		
DX3					.		
DX4					.		
DX5					.		
DX6					.		
DX7					.		
DX8					.		
DX9					.		
DX10					.		

ICD-9-CM CODES

PP1			.		
PR2			.		
PR3			.		
PR4			.		
PR5			.		
PR6			.		

INPATIENT RECORD

DISCHARGE SUMMARY—Patient 13 A

DATE OF ADMISSION: 4/24 **DATE OF DISCHARGE**: 4/27

DISCHARGE DIAGNOSIS: Stillborn infant; cephalopelvic disproportion; Cesarean section

ADMISSION HISTORY: Intrauterine term pregnancy with possible fetal death in utero
Cephalopelvic disproportion

COURSE IN HOSPITAL: The patient was admitted for induction of labor. She developed cephalopelvic disproportion and lack of established fetal heart tones for which a Cesarean section was undertaken. Unfortunately, the baby was stillborn at the time the Cesarean section was performed.

INSTRUCTIONS ON DISCHARGE: Continue with prenatal vitamins. Make an appointment with me in one week.

HISTORY AND PHYSICAL EXAMINATION—Patient 13 A

ADMITTED: 4/24

REASON FOR ADMISSION: Induction of labor

HISTORY OF PRESENT ILLNESS: Patient is a 29-year-old white female primigravida whose last menstrual period was last August and whose estimated date of confinement is April 7. She had a normal, uneventful pregnancy. She was seen for the first time in September. Sizes of dates were normal with the length of time. All her prenatal visits were normal. There was no evidence of hypertension although the patient was obese and she gained approximated 30 lb during the pregnancy. No proteinuria or sugar was noted in her urine and her hemoglobin remained stable throughout the pregnancy. Initial rubella titer showed immunity to German measles. No illnesses were noted during the pregnancy that were reported or required any treatment. She was admitted this a.m. with a history of not having felt the baby move for more than 24 hours. Heart tones were attempted to be elicited by the Doppler Fetone; however, no heart tones were noted by the nurse when she listened with the regular stethoscope. She thought she faintly heard normal heart tones. No fetal movements were noted by the nurse during labor. After the patient had no progress in labor for several hours, internal fetal monitor was applied to the vertex after the cervix was dilated and the membranes were ruptured by the physician. No fetal heart tones were picked up by the internal monitor either. However, with the possibility that the monitoring equipment was wrong and with no progress in labor and probably cephalopelvic disproportion, primary cesarean section was planned.

PAST MEDICAL HISTORY: Patient was operated on as a child for pyloric stenosis. Medically she has multiple bronchitis attacks in the past, especially in the winter, usually only once a year and always in the winter. No other medical problems and no other surgery are relevant. The blood type is B+.

ALLERGIES: None known

CHRONIC MEDICATIONS: None

PHYSICAL EXAMINATION: Well-developed, well-nourished obese white female admitted for induction of labor.

HEENT: Negative

LUNGS: Clear to P & A

HEART: Regular rhythm, no murmurs

BREASTS: No masses palpable

ABDOMEN: Full-term pregnancy, LOT position. Vertex is noted to be -1 station, cervix dilated to 4 cm. No edema or phlebitis of extremities. No fetal heart tones were detected at this time.

PROGRESS NOTES—Patient 13 A

DATE	**NOTE**
4/24	Admit to Labor and Delivery for decreased fetal heart tones and movement. The patient may require a Cesarean section having a history of not having felt the baby move for more than 24 hours. DATE: 4/24 PREOPERATIVE DX: Emergency Cesarean section POSTOPERATIVE DX: Stillborn infant; cephalopelvic disproportion
4/25	Patient doing well, appropriately grieving the loss of her baby. Referral given for support group. Incision clean and dry, no erythema.
4/26	Patient is voiding well, bowels moving, no infection.
4/27	Will discharge to home.

PHYSICIAN'S ORDERS—Patient 13 A

DATE	**ORDER**
4/24	Admit to labor and delivery monitor. Stat CBC Vaginal prep 1,000 cc lactated Ringer's solution Piggyback Pitocin 10 U in 500 cc D5LR at 6 cc per hour until contractions are 2 to 3 minutes apart and moderate in intensity Type and Screen Prepare for possible stat Cesarean section Postoperative orders: Tylenol with codeine Phosphate No. 3, 1 tablet every 4 hours p.r.n. × 4 days for pain. Dermoplast spray at bedside p.r.n. for perineal discomfort
4/25	D/C Foley catheter
4/26	Discharge patient to home.

OPERATIVE REPORT—Patient 13 A

DATE: 4/24

PREOPERATIVE DIAGNOSIS: Emergency Cesarean section

POSTOPERATIVE DIAGNOSIS: Stillborn infant; cephalopelvic disproportion

OPERATION: Classic Cesarean section

ANESTHESIA: General

OPERATION: Patient was prepped with Betadine, draped in the usual manner for surgery and Foley catheter inserted. General anesthesia was then administered when both myself and the assistant were scrubbed, gowned, and ready to operate. Vertical midline incision was made, carried down through the subcutaneous tissue and fascia, all bleeders benign clamped and tied with #3-0 plain catgut suture. Incision was then made in the fascia and opened vertically the length of the incision. Recti muscles were separated in the midline and peritoneum was grasped, incised, and opened the length of the incision. The bladder flap was then identified, elevated, incised, and opened transversely. Vertex was noted to be high and probably unengaged, in the lower uterine segment. Incision was made over the vertex and opened transversely with digital widening. The vertex was then easily delivered through the incision. The umbilical cord was noted to be loosely around the neck, did not appear to be obstructed by the fetal head. An 8-lb, 10-oz, pale, cyanotic stillborn infant was delivered. Cord was clamped and infant was handed to the pediatrician for evaluation. No amniotic fluid was noted in the uterus in the normal sense. There was some small amount of very thick pea-soup meconium. The placenta was manually removed from a normal fundal position. Uterus immediately tightened up. Pitocin was added to the intravenous line. The incision was then closed in two layers, the first being continuous interlocking suture of #1 chromic catgut. No bleeding was noted from the incision. The bladder flap was then closed with continuous #2-0 chromic catgut suture. All blood was removed from the pelvis. Incision was clean and no bleeding was noted. Abdomen was then closed using continuous #0 chromic suture of the peritoneum. Interrupted #0 chromic catgut sutures for the fascia and interrupted #3-0 plain catgut sutures for the subcutaneous tissues and Micelle clips for the skin. Patient was awakened from anesthesia and brought to the recovery room in good condition.

LABORATORY REPORTS—Patient 13 A

HEMATOLOGY

DATE: 4/24

Specimen	Results	Normal Values
WBC	5.0	4.3–11.0
RBC	4.7	4.5–5.9
HGB	13.6	13.5–17.5
HCT	42	41–52
MCV	90	80–100
MCHC	40	31–57
PLT	250	150–400

PATIENT 13 A

	ICD-9-CM CODES
PDX	
DX2	
DX3	
DX4	
DX5	
DX6	
DX7	
DX8	
DX9	
DX10	

	ICD-9-CM CODES
PP1	
PR2	
PR3	
PR4	
PR5	
PR6	

INPATIENT RECORD

DISCHARGE SUMMARY—Patient 14

DATE OF ADMISSION: 2/3 **DATE OF DISCHARGE**: 2/4

DISCHARGE DIAGNOSIS: Malignant ascites from metastatic adenocarcinoma of the colon

COURSE IN HOSPITAL: This 59-year-old white female patient was admitted for continuous infusion chemotherapy with 5-FU and Leucovoran. This was done under the care of Dr. ZXY. The patient tolerated her chemotherapy very well. She had no complications throughout her hospital course, and she was discharged to be followed further as an outpatient by her oncologist.

INSTRUCTIONS ON DISCHARGE: Follow up in the office.

HISTORY AND PHYSICAL EXAMINATION—Patient 14

ADMITTED: 2/3/200X

REASON FOR ADMISSION: Chemotherapy

HISTORY OF PRESENT ILLNESS: The patient is a 59-year-old white female with carcinomatosis and malignant ascites from colon carcinoma. She is admitted for continuous chemotherapy. The patient has a sigmoid colostomy and has had multiple abdominal surgeries for carcinoma, the first one was an anterior and posterior repair in 1982. She had six weeks of radiation therapy completed two years ago and has been on weekly chemotherapy consisting of 5-FU and methotrexate recently. Because of increasing abdominal girth, she was admitted in June 1987, and diagnosed with malignant ascites and carcinomatosis. At that time, she had an extensive evaluation including an upper gastrointestinal series, barium enema, CT scan, and ultrasound of the abdomen. She was told she had adhesions causing a partial obstruction. No further surgery was pursued. For the past week, she has complained of frequent vomiting. Her weight has decreased another six pounds. She denies any abdominal pain. She has occasional diarrhea for which she takes Questran. She has had no blood in her colostomy drainage.

PAST MEDICAL HISTORY: No hypertension, myocardial infarction, diabetes, or peptic ulcer disease. Anterior and posterior repair in 1982, colectomy, cholecystectomy, appendectomy, hysterectomy with bilateral salpingo-oophorectomy for uterine fibroids in 1968.

ALLERGIES: None

CHRONIC MEDICATIONS: Pancrease three times a day; Questran as needed for diarrhea; Os-Cal 2 × a day, 250 mg

FAMILY HISTORY: Mother died at age 80 years of old age. Father died of colon cancer at age 60 years.

SOCIAL HISTORY: Prior to that time, she smoked a pack a day for 20 years. She denies any alcohol intake. She works in the shipping department.

REVIEW OF SYSTEMS: Unremarkable

PHYSICAL EXAMINATION: An alert, white female in no acute distress

GENERAL APPEARANCE:

SKIN, HEAD, EYES, EARS, NOSE, THROAT: Pupils are equal, reactive to light and accommodation. Extraocular movements are intact. Fundi are benign. Tympanic membranes are normal.

MOUTH: No oral lesions are seen.

HEENT: Within normal limits

NECK: Carotids are plus 2 with no bruits. Thyroid is normal. There is no adenopathy at present.

LUNGS: Clear

HEART: Regular sinus rhythm. No murmur, rub, or gallop.

BREASTS: A small, approximately 3 mm, cystic lesion the medial aspect of her left breast at around eight o'clock. It is freely movable and nontender. There are no axillary nodes.

ABDOMEN: Distended. Sigmoid colostomy present. Right lower quadrant induration is present. There is no abdominal tenderness. There is no hepatosplenomegaly. Bowel sounds are normal.

PULSES: Femorals are plus 2 with no bruits. There are good pedal pulses bilaterally.

GENITALIA: Normal

RECTAL: Deferred

EXTREMITIES: No edema

NEUROLOGIC: Deep tendon reflexes are plus 2 throughout

LABORATORY DATA: Pending

IMPRESSION:

Abdominal carcinomatosis from colon cancer
Small left breast cyst

PLAN: The patient will be admitted for continuous chemotherapy.

PROGRESS NOTES—Patient 14

DATE	NOTE
2/3	Patient tolerating chemo well. No complaints offered.
2/4	Patient well hydrated, nausea and vomiting under control. Will discharge.

PHYSICIAN'S ORDERS—Patient 14

DATE	ORDER
2/3	Chemotherapy protocol in D5W Compazine 5 mg now, then Q4H prn
2/4	Discontinue IV Discharge the patient

PATIENT 14

ICD-9-CM CODES

PDX					.		
DX2					.		
DX3					.		
DX4					.		
DX5					.		
DX6					.		
DX7					.		
DX8					.		
DX9					.		
DX10					.		

ICD-9-CM CODES

PP1			.		
PR2			.		
PR3			.		
PR4			.		
PR5			.		
PR6			.		

INPATIENT RECORD

DISCHARGE SUMMARY—Patient 15

DATE OF ADMISSION: 1/3 **DATE OF DISCHARGE**: 1/7

DISCHARGE DIAGNOSIS: Recurrent carcinoma, left lung

This is a 63-year-old female who is two years status post left upper lobe resection for adenocarcinoma. Pathology at that time revealed a positive bronchial margin of resection. She was treated with postop radiation and has done extremely well. She has remained asymptotic with no postoperative difficulty. Follow up serial CT scans have revealed a new lesion in the apical portion of the left lung, which on needle biopsy was positive for adenocarcinoma. She was admitted specifically for a left thoracotomy and possible pneumonectomy.

PAST MEDICAL HISTORY: Positive for tobacco abuse 2 PPD × 30 years in the past. Significant for a right parotidectomy and also significant for hypertension, degenerative joint disease of lumbar spine, and chronic pulmonary disease. The patient also suffered a stroke in the left brain with resulting hemiparesis three years ago. Medications on discharge: Tenormin 25 mg once a day, Calan SR 240 mg twice a day, Moduretic one tablet q. day and K-Dur 10 meq q. day, Proventil MDI 2 puffs PO q.i.d. p.r.n., Azacort MDI 2 puffs PO t.i.d., Vioxx 25 mg PO daily.

PHYSICAL EXAMINATION: Revealed a well-healed right parotid incision. No supraclavicular adenopathy. She has a healed left posterior lateral thoracotomy scar. Impression is that of local recurrence, status post left upper lobectomy. She is to undergo a left pneumonectomy.

OPERATIVE FINDINGS AND HOSPITAL COURSE: There was a large mass in the remaining lung, extensive mediastinal fibrosis, bronchial margin free by frozen section. Following surgery she was placed in the intensive care unit postoperatively. The chest tube was removed on postoperative day number two.

She experienced some EKG changes consistent with acute nontransmural MI. Cardiology was consulted, and she was started on nitroglycerin and IV heparin. She was eventually weaned from her oxygen therapy.

She was started on regular diet and was discharged in good condition. Her wound was clean and dry.

INSTRUCTIONS ON DISCHARGE: Discharged home with instructions to follow up with cardiology next week. Also follow up with me in the office.

HISTORY AND PHYSICAL EXAMINATION—Patient 15

Admitted: 1/3

HISTORY OF PRESENT ILLNESS: Patient is a 63-year-old right-handed female with history of recurrent adenocarcinoma of apical segment of left upper lobe of lung. She has received radiation therapy to her chest. She weighs 123 pounds. She also has chronic obstructive pulmonary disease.

REVIEW OF SYSTEMS: She can climb two flights of steps with minimal difficulties. She has a significant underbite. She has stiffness in lower spine, worse in the a.m. She has hypertension and took her Tenormin 25 mg, Calan SR 240 mg this a.m.

PAST SURGICAL HISTORY: She had a right parotidectomy seven years ago and was told they needed to use a "very small" ETT. Two years ago she underwent a left upper lobe resection at this facility. Previous medical records are being requested.

ALLERGIES: She is allergic to sulfa. Postoperatively last time she received Demerol. She also had hallucinations in the ICU for several days. She blames the hallucinations on the Demerol. The only allergy sign was hallucinations.

PHYSICAL EXAMINATION: Revealed a well healed right parotid incision. No supraclavicular adenopathy. She has a healed left posterior lateral thoracotomy scar. Impression is that of local recurrence, status post left upper lobectomy. She is to undergo a left completion pneumonectomy, muscle flap coverage of bronchial stump. The patient has hemiparesis in the right extremities.

IMPRESSION: Recurrent carcinoma left lower lobe of lung

PLAN: Pneumonectomy of left lung. The patient is agreeable to general endotracheal anesthesia or the use of epidural narcotic. She is agreeable to postoperative ventilation if necessary.

PROGRESS NOTES—Patient 15

DATE	NOTE
1/3	Attending Physician: Admit for recurrent lung carcinoma, s/p radiation therapy. Consent signed for pneumonectomy. Epidural morphine usage postop explained to and discussed with the patient. She is agreeable. **Anesthesia Preop**: Patient evaluated and examined. General anesthesia chosen. Patient agrees. Will provide postop epidural morphine for pain management s/p thoracotomy. Attending Physician: **Procedure Note**: **Preop Dx**: Local recurrence of carcinoma of the lung **Postop Dx**: Same **Procedure**: Pneumonectomy with muscle flap coverage of bronchial stump Complications: R/O Intraop MI **Anesthesia Postop**: Patient in stable condition following GEA with possible intraoperative MI due to hypotension. CPK to be evaluated as available. Patient comfortable with epidural morphine. No adverse effects of anesthesia experienced.

1/4 Attending Physician:
Path report confirms recurrent adenocarcinoma. Patient stable but with persistent hypotension resolving slowly—will consult cardiology. CPK MB positive. Incision clean and dry. COPD stable, arthritis stable.

Cardiology Consult:
The patient has resolving intraoperative myocardial infarction. Will continue to monitor.

1/5 Attending Physician:
Looks and feels well, weaning off morphine. Blood pressure stable. Left pleural space expanding and filling space. Chest tube removed, epidural cath removed.

Cardiology Consult:
The patient looking and feeling better.

1/6 Attending Physician:
Patient stable for discharge in a.m. Cardiology to follow.

OPERATIVE REPORT—Patient 15

DATE: 1/3

OPERATION: Pneumonectomy

PREOPERATIVE DIAGNOSIS: Recurrent carcinoma of left lung

POSTOPERATIVE DIAGNOSIS: Same

ANESTHESIA: General endotracheal anesthesia

OPERATIVE FINDINGS: There was a large mass in the left lower lobe.

The patient was prepped and draped in the usual fashion. Following thoracotomy the left lung was completely removed. A muscle flap coverage was used for the bronchial stump. During the procedure the patient experienced an episode of hypotension, watch for resulting MI. The patient was fluid resuscitated and sent to the recovery room in good condition.

PATHOLOGY REPORT—Patient 15

DATE: 1/3

SPECIMEN: Left lung, resected

CLINICAL DATA: This is a 63-year-old female with recurrent disease on CT scan

DIAGNOSIS: Adenocarcinoma of the apical portion of the lung, bronchial margin is free of disease

PHYSICIAN'S ORDERS—Patient 15

DATE	ORDER
1/3	Admit to surgical floor Standard orders for thoracotomy Tenormin 25 mg q.d. Calan SR 240 mg twice a day Moduretic one tab. q.d K-Dur 10 meq q.d. in a.m. Vioxx 25 mg PO daily in a.m. Proventil (albuterol) MDI 2 puffs PO q.i.d. Azmacort MDI 2 puffs PO q.i.d. CBC Postop orders: Admit to ICU Serial CPK stat CBC SMA 12 Anesthesia: Morphine pump ad lib D5nss 100 cc/hr Strict input and output documentation
1/4	Attending MD: Consult Cardiology Cardiology: Lasix 20 mg b.i.d. PO D/C IV
1/5	Transfer to floor Continue meds
1/6	Discharge patient in a.m.

LABORATORY REPORTS—Patient 15

HEMATOLOGY

DATE: 1/3

Specimen	Results	Normal Values
WBC	5.7	4.3–11.0
RBC	5.0	4.5–5.9
HGB	15.6	13.5–17.5
HCT	47	41–52
MCV	89	80–100
MCHC	42	31–57
PLT	300	150–400

HEMATOLOGY

DATE: 1/4

Specimen	Results	Normal Values
WBC	5.6	4.3–11.0
RBC	4.0 L	4.5–5.9
HGB	13.4 L	13.5–17.5
HCT	40 L	41–52
MCV	82	80–100
MCHC	33	31–57
PLT	200	150–400

LABORATORY REPORT—Patient 15

CHEMISTRY

DATE: 1/3

Specimen	Results	Normal Values
GLUC	90	70–110
BUN	27 H	8–25
CREAT	1.0	0.5–1.5
NA	138	136–146
K	4.0	3.5–5.5
CL	100	95–110
CO2	28	24–32
CA	8.9	8.4–10.5
PHOS	2.9	2.5–4.4
MG	2.0	1.6–3.0
T BILI	1.0	0.2–1.2
D BILI	0.04	0.0–0.5
PROTEIN	7.0	6.0–8.0
ALBUMIN	5.3	5.0–5.5
AST	35	0–40
ALT	50	30–65
GGT		15–85
LD		100–190
ALK PHOS		50–136
URIC ACID		2.2–7.7
MB	7 H, 15 H, 12 H, 9 H	0–5.0
CPK	221 , 250 H, 275 H, 230	21–232

RADIOLOGY REPORT—Patient 15

DATE: 1/3

Chest x-ray: Reveals mass in the left lower lobe. There are surgical clips in the thorax from apparent previous surgery. The thoracic organs are midline and the vasculature is normal.

IMPRESSION: Carcinoma LLL, no congestive heart failure.

RADIOLOGY REPORT—Patient 15

DATE: 1/4

Chest x-ray: Reveals absence of left lung. Other architecture is normal other than post-operative changes. The thoracic organs are midline and the vasculature is normal.

IMPRESSION: Postop changes consistent with lobectomy, no congestive heart failure.

EKG REPORT—Patient 15

DATE: 1/3

Normal sinus rhythm

DATE: 1/4

There are nonspecific ST changes consistent with possible evolving myocardial infarction

DATE: 1/5

Possible acute myocardial infarction, please correlate with other clinical findings.

PATIENT 15

	ICD-9-CM CODES						
PDX					.		
DX2					.		
DX3					.		
DX4					.		
DX5					.		
DX6					.		
DX7					.		
DX8					.		
DX9					.		
DX10					.		

	ICD-9-CM CODES				
PP1			.		
PR2			.		
PR3			.		
PR4			.		
PR5			.		
PR6			.		

INPATIENT RECORD

DISCHARGE SUMMARY—Patient 16

DATE OF ADMISSION: 4/19 **DATE OF DISCHARGE**: 4/24

DISCHARGE DIAGNOSIS:

Acute myocardial infarction
Hyperlipidemia
Complete heart block
Upper gastrointestinal hemorrhage
Arteriosclerotic heart disease

ADMISSION HISTORY: This is a 45-year-old white male with a history of hyperlipidemia and tobacco use. He presented to the hospital with an acute myocardial infarction. He was treated with intravenous TPA and had a reperfusion. The patient continued to have chest pain with an inferior ST elevation on EKG.

COURSE IN HOSPITAL: The patient sustained an acute myocardial infarction. The patient presented with an acute myocardial infarction and underwent catheterization. The patient was found to have stenosis of the mid right coronary artery and right distal coronary artery. The left coronary branches have minimal noncritical disease. The left ventricular ejection fraction was approximately 45% with inferior wall hypokinesis.

The patient had a successful stent PTCA to the mid-RCA with a stent. I initially attempted to dilate with a balloon, but the results were inadequate and proceeded to place a 4.0-mm J&J stent. The patient continued to have anginal symptomatology and for this reason was taken to the OR for CABG × 2. He did well after the CABG × 2 without any anginal symptoms.

The patient also had gastrointestinal bleeding following the PTCA. The patient developed retching and hematemesis and anemia for which he required blood transfusion. The probable cause of the nausea and vomiting was a reaction to anesthesia. Upper endoscopy revealed no evidence of peptic ulcer disease.

At the present time the patient has been treated with Aspirin and Ticlid and has been doing very well. The plan is to discharge him home with follow up in my office next week.

INSTRUCTIONS ON DISCHARGE: Follow up in 1 week in my office next week. Medications include; Aspirin 1 tablet per day, Ticlid 250 mg twice per day, Tagamet 400 mg twice per day and sublingual nitroglycerin as needed for chest pain. Condition upon discharge is stable. Activity is restricted until cardiac rehabilitation.

HISTORY AND PHYSICAL EXAMINATION—Patient 16

ADMITTED: 4/19

Acute myocardial infarction
Complete heart block
Ventricular ectopy
Possible ASHD

REASON FOR ADMISSION: Pain in chest

HISTORY OF PRESENT ILLNESS: This is a pleasant 45-year-old male with a history of hyperlipidemia and previous tobacco use. He also has a family history of coronary artery disease. He denies any prior history of coronary artery disease, myocardial infarction, or CVAs. The patient has been essentially very healthy, except for occasional skipped heartbeat in the past for which he has never taken any medications. The patient is presently on no medications.

Two days ago, he started complaining of a dull chest ache that appeared to radiate to his left arm and lasted for a few minutes. He was brought to the emergency department and was noted to have an acute inferior myocardial infarction with complete heart block. I was consulted to evaluate the patient and proceeded with administration of TPA therapy and IV Atropine for complete heart block. At the present time the patient is in sinus rhythm and is presently receiving IV TPA. He denies any melena, hematochezia. Denies any shortness of breath, PND, orthopnea.

PAST MEDICAL HISTORY: He denies any history of hypertension or diabetes. He has a history of high cholesterol. He states that he had his cholesterol checked approximately 3 months ago and it was around 310. He used to smoke tobacco, one pack a day for 20 years. He quit smoking 6 months ago. He denies any history of coronary artery disease, myocardial infarction, or cerebrovascular accident.

He has a history of heart palpitations that he describes as skipped heartbeat in the past for which he is not taking any medications. He has never had an evaluation.

He has a history of kidney stones two years ago. He denies any history of peptic ulcer disease. He has a history of hemorrhoidal bleeding in the past. The last episode of bleeding was 6 or 7 months ago.

The patient denies any trauma or recent surgery.

ALLERGIES: Patient has no known drug allergies.

CHRONIC MEDICATIONS: None

SOCIAL HISTORY: He quit tobacco 6 months ago and denies alcohol abuse. He is a construction worker.

REVIEW OF SYSTEMS: Denies melena, hematochezia, hematemesis and he denies change in weight.

PHYSICAL EXAMINATION: This is a pleasant gentleman who appears slightly diaphoretic and is expressing having mild chest pain which is better from admission. He is presently receiving IV TPA. Vital signs are as follows: Blood pressure is 100/70; heart rate in the 80s. The neck shows no JVD, no carotid bruits. The lungs are clear and heart is regular rate with S4 gallop rhythm and no murmurs. The abdomen is soft and nontender. Extremities show no edema. The pulses of his femoral and dorsalis pedis are 2+ bilaterally. Neurological examination reveals an alert and oriented male × 3.

LABORATORY DATA: SMA-7, Sodium 138, potassium 3.7, BUN 7, creatinine 0.9. CBC showed a white blood cell count of 12. Hematocrit 37, hemoglobin 13. Platelet count is 312. His EKG showed complete heart block with significant ST elevation in the inferior leads with reciprocal changes in the anteroseptal leads, consistent with an acute inferior wall myocardial infarction. His chest x-ray is pending.

IMPRESSION AND PLAN: Acute myocardial infarction that appears to have started around 10:30 in the morning. He presented very early to the emergency department and was treated aggressively with intravenous TPA, intravenous aspirin, intravenous nitroglycerin.

We will continue the TPA and begin lidocaine. We will obtain cardiac enzymes and admit to CCU. The patient will need cardiac catheterization evaluated within 48 hours. If symptoms recur or patient does not have evidence of reperfusion will need urgent cardiac catheterization. If heart block occurs will treat with intravenous Atropine on a p.r.n. basis. We will check a cholesterol and lipid profile in the hospital.

CONSULTATION—Patient 16

DATE: 4/20

CHIEF COMPLAINT: Vomiting blood

REVIEW OF SYSTEMS: This 45-year-old white male was seen in consultation because of GI bleeding. The patient was admitted one day ago with acute myocardial infarction. He was treated with TPA and later went to cardiac catheterization where he was found to have a lesion of the mid RCA and distal RCA. Today the patient exhibited hematemesis with retching. He has no past history of ulcer disease or GI bleeding.

PHYSICAL EXAMINATION: Physical examination reveals an adult male lying in bed. Blood pressure is 120/80, pulses 60. HEENT: Pale. LUNGS: Clear. HEART: Regular rate and rhythm. ABDOMEN: Benign.

LABORATORY: WBC is 12, hemoglobin 12, and hematocrit 37

IMPRESSION: Upper GI bleeding; rule out ulcer disease

RECOMMENDATION: We will perform an upper endoscopy to be performed today after informed consent is obtained. Further recommendations are to follow.

PROGRESS NOTES—Patient 16

DATE	NOTE
4/19	This is a 45-year-old white male with a history of increased cholesterol, no prior coronary artery disease, MI or CVA. He presented with acute ischemia and heart block. He was given IV TPA; 1–1½ hours after TPA he had severe chest pain with elevated ST inferior leads. He was treated emergently for urgent catheter and PTCA. Post Catheter/Stent Procedure: Left heart catheter, coronary angio, left ventricular angiography Results: Normal LCA, 99% mid-RCA and 70 stenosis distal RCA, successful stent PTCA to mid RCA with excellent results.
4/20	Cardiac: Patient continues to have pain. Will prepare for CABG when patient stable from GI perspective. GI: The patient experienced vomiting with flecks of blood after the cardiac catheterization. In light of apparent acute blood loss anemia will check for peptic ulcer. Probable reaction to anesthetics. Endoscopy Note: Preop: Gastrointestinal bleeding Postop: Gastrointestinal bleeding, etiology unknown Procedure: EGD Complications: None
4/21	Patient is scheduled for the OR today. Bleeding stable. OP Note: Preop: Critical stenosis of the mid-RCA and distal RCA Postop: Same Operation: CABG × 2 Complications: None
4/22	Patient recovering well. No chest pain or shortness of breath. The wound looks good. Will monitor blood loss anemia. The patient declines blood transfusion.
4/23	Chest clear, no chest pain, abdomen is soft with bowel sounds. Will transfer to the floor.
4/24	Wound healing well, patient OOB ambulating, no chest pain, lungs clear.
4/25	Will discharge today. Patient to follow up in 1 week.

PHYSICIAN'S ORDERS—Patient 16

DATE	ORDER
4/19	3/19 Admit to CCU DX: Acute MI Cardiac enzymes q. 8 hours × 3 CBC q. day × 3 Meds: IV nitro @ 20 ug/min

	ASA 325 mg PO q. day Ticlid 250 mg PO b.i.d. Xanax 0.25 mg PO t.i.d. p.r.n. Restoril 30 mgs PO q. h p.r.n. for sleep Zantac 150 mg PO b.i.d. daily PT and INR, PTT Diet: cardiac Vital signs q. 15 min × 8 then q.i.d. Bed rest O_2 at 2 L/min. NS at 150 cc/hr for 10 hours
4/20	Lopressor 25 mg PO t.i.d. Social worker consult re: payment issues CBC at 6 p.m. NPO for now Possible endoscopy Postendoscopy orders Watch VS Resume previous orders No heparin or TPA Hgb and Hct q. 6 h NS at 125 cc/hr D/C ASA, Ticlid for now Tagamet drip per protocol
4/21	Postop CABG Orders: Continue present ventilator settings Daily Electrolytes and CBC Morphine sulfate 15 mg PO q. 4h p.r.n. TED stockings Weigh patient daily Routine weaning in a.m. Lidocaine 3 g/min Continue Tagamet drip
4/22	Decrease Lidocaine to 2 g/min Extubate patient as soon as weaned from ventilator Chest tubes to low suction Oxygen face mask 4 L/min Encourage incentive spirometry
4/23	Nutrition consult re: low fat, low salt diet D/C Tagamet drip to 250 mg q. 6 Benadryl prn for sleep Consult cardiac rehab
4/24	D/C oxygen Consult home healthcare for postsurgical monitoring
4/25	Discharge patient

OPERATIVE REPORT—Patient 16

DATE: 4/21

PREOPERATIVE DIAGNOSIS: Critical stenosis of mid right coronary artery and distal right coronary artery

POSTOPERATIVE DIAGNOSIS: Same

OPERATION: Coronary bypass × 2 using saphenous vein from aorta to right mid coronary artery and distal right coronary artery

ANESTHESIA: General

Under general anesthesia with arterial and pulmonary artery monitoring with sterile prep and drape, a sterile midline sternotomy was performed. The pericardium was opened. Purse-string sutures were placed in the ascending aorta and the right atrium. Extracorporeal circulation was undertaken at this point. The saphenous vein was harvested from the right leg in the usual fashion. The patient was then placed on cardiopulmonary bypass. Cardioplegia was affected. The right coronary artery was dissected. Using a 6-0 Prolene suture an end-to-side anastomosis was created between the right mid coronary artery and the aorta. A second opening for end to side anastomosis was performed from the aorta to the distal right coronary artery. Following spontaneous contraction of the heart the patient was removed from cardiopulmonary bypass. Approximating the pericardium then began closure. Hemostasis was obtained. The sternum was approximated with a parasternal wire and fascia and skin with vicryl. The patient tolerated the procedure well and was transferred to the recovery room in stable condition.

ENDOSCOPY REPORT—Patient 16

DATE: 4/20

Pre-gastrointestinal bleeding; rule out ulcers

Post-upper gastrointestinal bleeding; stomach and duodenum appear unremarkable

MEDS: Demerol 50 mg IV
Versed 3 mg IV

PROCEDURE: Esophagogastroduodenoscopy

The patient was sedated and the scope inserted into the hypopharynx. There was fresh blood oozing from an area in the hiatal hernia pouch just below the gastroesophageal junction. The scope was passed further down to visualize the remainder of the stomach and the duodenum. All areas appeared unremarkable with no other ulcers or lesions identified. The patient tolerated the procedure well. He did have some retching and vomiting after the scope was removed.

CARDIAC CATHERIZATION SUMMARY—Patient 16

DATE: 4/19

PROCEDURE:

Left heart catheterization
Left ventricular angiography
Coronary angiography
Stent to mid right coronary artery

After obtaining informed consent the patient was taken to the cardiac catheterization laboratory. He was prepped and draped in the usual fashion and 2% Xylocaine was used to anesthetize the right groin. 6-French sheaths were introduced into the right femoral artery and vein and a 6-French multipurpose catheter was used for left heart catheterization, coronary angiography and left ventricular angiography. I then proceeded to perform a Stent/PTCA to the mid RCA. A HTF wire was used to cross the RCA stenosis and a 4.0-mm J&J Stent was placed in the mid right coronary artery with excellent results. The final angiogram was obtained and the guiding catheterization was removed. The sheaths were securely sutured and the patient tolerated the procedure well without complications.

FINDINGS:

1. Left heart catheterization revealed an elevated resting left ventricular end-diastolic pressure of 18 mm Hg.
2. Left ventricular angiography revealed mild to moderate inferior wall hypokinesis with overall mildly depressed left ventricular systolic function and an estimated global ejection fraction of 45%.
3. Coronary angiography (using single catheter): The left coronary artery arises normally from the left sinus of Valsalva. The left main artery, left anterior descending coronary artery and its branches, and the circumflex artery and its branches have minimal irregularities.

The right coronary artery arises normally from the right sinus of Valsalva. There is a 99% very eccentric stenosis in the large mid right coronary artery and a 70% stenosis of the distal right coronary artery.

IMPRESSION: Arteriosclerotic coronary artery disease was found. There was a successful implantation of 4.0-mm J&J stent in the mid right coronary artery. This site was predilated with a 4.0-mm balloon, then followed by the insertion of a stent.

The mid right coronary artery shows excellent results. Pending the patient's progress we may have to proceed with CABG. The patient will remain on aspirin, Coumadin, and nitrates in the hospital. He will remain on intravenous heparin while his PT levels are adjusted.

LABORATORY REPORTS—Patient 16

HEMATOLOGY

DATE: 4/19

Specimen	Results	Normal Values
WBC	9.3	4.3–11.0
RBC	4.4 L	4.5–5.9
HGB	12.7 L	13.5–17.5
HCT	41	41–52
MCV	89	80–100
MCHC	33.9	31–57
PLT	Adequate	

HEMATOLOGY

DATE: 4/20

Specimen	Results	Normal Values
WBC	7.7	4.3–11.0
RBC	4.4 L	4.5–5.9
HGB	12.0 L	13.5–17.5
HCT	41	41–52
MCV	89.6	80–100
MCHC	33.9	31–57
PLT	Adequate	

HEMATOLOGY

DATE: 4/21

Specimen	Results	Normal Values
WBC	08.0	4.3–11.0
RBC	2.88 L	4.5–5.9
HGB	8.6 L	13.5–17.5
HCT	25.8 L	41–52
MCV	89	80–100
MCHC	33.9	31–57
PLT	Adequate	

HEMATOLOGY

DATE: 4/21

Specimen	Results	Normal Values
WBC	08.0	4.3–11.0
RBC	4.5	4.5–5.9
HGB	9.0 L	13.5–17.5
HCT	26.5 L	41–52
MCV	89	80–100
MCHC	33.9	31–57
PLT	Adequate	

HEMATOLOGY

DATE: 4/21

Specimen	Results	Normal Values
WBC	08.0	4.3–11.0
RBC	4.5	4.5–5.9
HGB	9.3 L	13.5–17.5
HCT	27.3 L	41–52
MCV	89	80–100
MCHC	33.9	31–57
PLT	Adequate	

HEMATOLOGY

DATE: 4/22

Specimen	Results	Normal Values
WBC	7.0	4.3–11.0
RBC	2.95 L	4.5–5.9
HGB	9.0 L	13.5–17.5
HCT	26.3 L	41–52
MCV	89	80–100
MCHC	33.9	31–57
PLT	Adequate	

HEMATOLOGY

DATE: 4/23

Specimen	Results	Normal Values
WBC	6.7	4.3–11.0
RBC	2.78 L	4.5–5.9
HGB	8.4 L	13.5–17.5
HCT	24.8 L	41–52
MCV	89.2	80–100
MCHC	34	31–57
PLT	Adequate	

HEMATOLOGY

DATE: 4/24

Specimen	Results	Normal Values
WBC	8.0	4.3–11.0
RBC	4.3 L	4.5–5.9
HGB	9.2 L	13.5–17.5
HCT	27.0 L	41–52
MCV	89	80–100
MCHC	33.9	31–57
PLT	Adequate	

HEMATOLOGY

DATE: 4/25

Specimen	Results	Normal Values
WBC	08.0	4.3–11.0
RBC	4.5	4.5–5.9
HGB	11.1 L	13.5–17.5
HCT	32 L	41–52
MCV	89	80–100
MCHC	33.9	31–57
PLT	Adequate	

LABORATORY REPORTS—Patient 16

CHEMISTRY

DATE: 4/19

Specimen	Results	Normal Values
GLUC	97	70–110
BUN	12	8–25
CREAT	1.0	0.5–1.5
NA	134 L	136–146
K	4.0	3.5–5.5
CL	109	95–110
CO2	33 H	24–32
CA	9.1	8.4–10.5
PHOS	3.0	2.5–4.4
MG	2.0	1.6–3.0
CK	1702 H	26–221
LD	327 H	106–210
CK MB	93.7 H	0.0–4.4
Relative Index	5.5	
AST	36	0–40
ALT	44	30–65
GCT	70	15–85
LD	110	100–190
ALK PHOS	114	50–136
URIC ACID	6.0	2.2–7.7
CHOL	275 H	0–200
TRIG	140	10–160

CHEMISTRY

DATE: 4/20

Specimen	**Results**	**Normal Values**
GLUC	97	70–110
BUN	12	8–25
CREAT	1.0	0.5–1.5
NA	134 L	136–146
K	5.6 H	3.5–5.5
CL	109	95–110
CO2	33 H	24–32
CA	9.1	8.4–10.5
PHOS	3.0	2.5–4.4
MG	2.0	1.6–3.0
CK	1277 H	26–221
LD	345 H	106–210
CK MB	68.7 H	0.0–4.4
Relative Index	5.4	
AST	36	0–40
ALT	44	30–65
GCT	70	15–85
LD	110	100–190
ALK PHOS	114	50–136
URIC ACID	6.0	2.2–7.7
CHOL	275 H	0–200
TRIG	140	10–160

CHEMISTRY

DATE: 4/21

Specimen	**Results**	**Normal Values**
GLUC	97	70–110
BUN	12	8–25
CREAT	1.0	0.5–1.5
NA	134 L	136–146
K	5.6 H	3.5–5.5
CL	109	95–110
CO2	33 H	24–32
CA	9.1	8.4–10.5
PHOS	3.0	2.5–4.4
MG	2.0	1.6–3.0
CK	1024 H	26–221
LD	372 H	106–210
CK MB	40.3 H	0.0–4.4
Relative Index	3.9	
AST	36	0–40
ALT	44	30–65
GCT	70	15–85
LD	110	100–190
ALK PHOS	114	50–136
URIC ACID	6.0	2.2–7.7
CHOL	275 H	0–200
TRIG	140	10–160

RADIOLOGY REPORT—Patient 16

DATE: 4/19

CHEST, SUPINE: There is no gross evidence of acute inflammatory disease or congestive heart failure.

IMPRESSION: No acute disease

RADIOLOGY REPORT—Patient 16

DATE: 4/21

DIAGNOSIS: The patient appears to have undergone sternotomy. The heart appears normal. The endotracheal tube is in place as is the Swan-Ganz catheter.

IMPRESSION: Stable postoperative chest

EKG REPORT—Patient 16

DATE: 4/19

IMPRESSION: Elevated ST changes. Cannot eliminate the possibility of ischemia. Complete heart block is also noted.

EKG REPORT—Patient 16

DATE: 4/20

IMPRESSION: Acute inferior myocardial infarction. Complete heart block has resolved.

PATIENT 16

ICD-9-CM CODES

PDX					.		
DX2					.		
DX3					.		
DX4					.		
DX5					.		
DX6					.		
DX7					.		
DX8					.		
DX9					.		
DX10					.		

ICD-9-CM CODES

PP1			.		
PR2			.		
PR3			.		
PR4			.		
PR5			.		
PR6			.		

INPATIENT RECORD

DISCHARGE SUMMARY—Patient 17

DATE OF ADMISSION: 9/8 **DATE OF DISCHARGE**: 9/10

DISCHARGE DIAGNOSIS:

1. Acute pyelonephritis
2. Septicemia, resistant to ampicillin and penicillin

ADMISSION HISTORY: This 21-year-old female was admitted to the hospital with discomfort in the right side. Other than this she has been healthy. On the day of admission she developed severe discomfort in the lower back. She was having fever and chills for which she took an aspirin and then she came to the emergency department.

COURSE IN HOSPITAL: The patient was treated with intravenous antibiotics in the form of gentamicin and cefoxitin. She continued to improve on this regimen and became afebrile after about three days of treatment. Her physical examination remained essentially unchanged; however, there was marked improvement in the patient's general condition. The patient also had an onset of herpes simplex infection on her upper lip, for which she was given Zovirax ointment.

INSTRUCTIONS ON DISCHARGE: The patient was discharged home on ciprofloxacin 500 mg po bid × 12 days. A repeat blood culture done just prior to discharge showed no growth at the end of 7 days. She is to be followed up in my office in about a week after discharge to have a repeat urine culture done. The patient was also given a prescription for Zyban to assist smoking cessation.

HISTORY AND PHYSICAL EXAMINATION—Patient 17

ADMITTED: 9/8

REASON FOR ADMISSION: This was the first hospital admission for this 21-year-old white female, who experienced difficulty about 3 days prior to admission. This was in the form of discomfort in the right side of the lower back and also some dysuria. On the evening of admission, she started experiencing some fever and chills and took some aspirin. This did not help her and she came to the emergency department.

HISTORY OF PRESENT ILLNESS:

PAST MEDICAL HISTORY: Remarkable only for "walking pneumonia" treated with erythromycin 3 months ago. She also suffered contusion of her right kidney after a fall from a horse about 4 years prior to admission.

ALLERGIES: None known

CHRONIC MEDICATIONS: None

FAMILY HISTORY: Remarkable for multiple members of the family having diabetes mellitus.

SOCIAL HISTORY: The patient lives with two friends and is employed by a saddle shop. She drinks about one drink a week and smokes a pack of cigarettes a day.

REVIEW OF SYSTEMS: The patient relates that there has been no weight gain or loss and that she was well functioning until three days ago when she developed lower back pain, primarily on the right side. She also relates that she has had dysuria for this same time period.

PHYSICAL EXAMINATION: On admission, significant for temperature of 103 degrees; pulse 120 beats per minute, regular; blood pressure 120/70; respirations 16.

VITAL SIGNS: P 120/min, regular; BP 120/70; Temp 103 degrees; R 16/min, regular.

GENERAL: The patient is a well-developed female of her stated age. She appears lethargic but responsive. The patient appears septic.

SKIN: Warm to touch

HEENT: Pupils equal, react briskly to light. Mucous membranes of the eyes, nose, mouth, and oropharynx are normal.

NECK: Supple, trachea is central, the carotid pulses are symmetrical. There is no goiter.

LUNGS: Clear to auscultation and percussion

BACK: Positive pain to palpation and percussion right costovertebral angle

HEART: Peripheral pulses are symmetrical. The cardiac apex is not displaced. The heart sounds are normal and there are no added sounds or murmurs.

ABDOMEN: Soft, nontender, with no masses palpable. The bowel sounds are normal.

GENITALIA: Normal female

RECTAL: Deferred

EXTREMITIES: Femoral pulses normal, no edema

NEUROLOGIC: Grossly intact

LABORATORY DATA: WBC 15.9 with differential of 57 Segs; 33 Bands; 6 Lymphs; 4 Monos. Electrolytes were normal. BUN 11. Urine culture grew out *E coli,* more than 100,000 colonies per mL. Blood culture was also positive for *E coli.* This was sensitive to gentamicin and cefoxitin, as well as many other antibiotics. Urinalysis on admission revealed many WBCs and marked bacteriuria. Chest x-ray was unremarkable.

IMPRESSION: Admit for clinical features of acute pyelonephritis and septicemia

PLAN: Hydrate and start IV antibiotics

PROGRESS NOTES—Patient 17

DATE	NOTE
9/8	Patient admitted for evaluation of flank pain and fever. She also has a lesion on her lip. This appears to be herpes simplex. Will treat infection process with antibiotics following obtaining cultures. Will monitor her renal function.
9/10	The patient's fever decreasing. Patient comfortable and tolerating antibiotics. Will continue IVs. The importance of stopping cigarette use was discussed with the patient. She is willing to quit and she will be given a prescription for Zyban at discharge.
9/11	Patient is afebrile today. Will discharge when able to obtain transportation.

PHYSICIAN'S ORDERS—Patient 17

DATE	ORDER
9/8	Admit to floor for evaluation of febrile illness Urinalysis CBC and SMA 16 Urine culture and sensitivity Blood cultures × 2 Chest x-ray Pyelogram D5W 125 cc/h × 3 Strict input and output Zovirax ointment prn to lip Gentamicin 80 mg IV q. 8 H × 3d Cefoxitin 1 g IV q. 8 H × 3 days
9/9	D5W 100 cc/ph
9/10	Discharge patient when transportation is arranged Ciprofloxacin 500 mg po b.i.d. × 12 days Zyban 150 mg PO daily × 3 days then b.i.d. Follow up in the office in 1 week

LABORATORY REPORTS—Patient 17

HEMATOLOGY

DATE: 9/8

Specimen	Results	Normal Values
WBC	15.9 H	4.3–11.0
RBC	5.5	4.5–5.9
HGB	14.0	13.5–17.5
HCT	45	41–52
MCV	90	80–100
MCHC	41	31–57
PLT	251	150–400

CHEMISTRY

DATE: 9/8

Specimen	Results	Normal Values
GLUC	100	70–110
BUN	11	8–25
CREAT	1.0	0.5–1.5
NA	143	136–146
K	4.0	3.5–5.5
CL	98	95–110
CO2	30	24–32
CA	9.0	8.4–10.5
PHOS	3.0	2.5–4.4
MG	2.0	1.6–3.0
T BILI	1.0	0.2–1.2
D BILI	0.3	0.0–0.5
PROTEIN	7.0	6.0–8.0
ALBUMIN	5.2	5.0–5.5
AST	25	0–40
ALT	40	30–65
GGT	60	15–85
LD		100–190
ALK PHOS		50–136
URIC ACID		2.2–7.7
CHOL		0–200
TRIG		10–160

URINALYSIS

DATE: 9/8

Test	Result	Ref Range
SP GRAVITY	1.03	1.005–1.035
PH	6	5–7
PROT	NEG	NEG
GLUC	NEG	NEG
KETONES	NEG	NEG
BILI	NEG	NEG
BLOOD	NEG	NEG
LEU EST	POS	NEG
NITRATES	POS	NEG
RED SUBS	NEG	NEG

MICROBIOLOGY

DATE	TEST TYPE: Culture and Sensitivity	
9/8	SOURCE: Urine	
	SITE:	
	GRAM STAIN RESULTS	
	CULTURE RESULTS: E.coli, 100,000/ml	
	SUSCEPTIBILITY:	
9/10	AMPICILLIN	R
	CEFAZOLIN	S
	CEFOTAXIME	S
	CEFTRIAXONE	S
	CEFUROXIME	S
	CEPHALOTHIN	S
	CIPROFLOXACIN	S
	ERYTHROMYCIN	S
	GENTAMICIN	S
	OXACILLIN	S
	PENICILLIN	R
	PIPERACILLIN	
	TETRACYCLINE	
	TOBRAMYCIN	
	TRIMETH/SULF	
	VANCOMYCIN	

S = SUSCEPTIBLE
R = RESISTANT
I = INTERMEDIATE
M = MODERATELY SUSCEP

LABORATORY RESULTS—Patient 17

DATE: 9/11

URINE CULTURE: No growth for 24 hours

MICROBIOLOGY

DATE	TEST TYPE:	
9/8	Culture and Sensitivity #1	
	SOURCE: Blood	
	SITE:	
	GRAM STAIN RESULTS	
	CULTURE RESULTS: E. coli	
	SUSCEPTIBILITY:	
9/10	AMPICILLIN	R
	CEFAZOLIN	S
	CEFOTAXIME	S
	CEFTRIAXONE	S
	CEFUROXIME	S
	CEPHALOTHIN	S
	CIPROFLOXACIN	S
	ERYTHROMYCIN	S
	GENTAMICIN	S
	OXACILLIN	S
	PENICILLIN	R
	PIPERACILLIN	
	TETRACYCLINE	
	TOBRAMYCIN	
	TRIMETH/SULF	
	VANCOMYCIN	

S = SUSCEPTIBLE
R = RESISTANT
I = INTERMEDIATE
M = MODERATELY SUSCEP

MICROBIOLOGY

DATE	TEST TYPE:	
9/8	Culture and Sensitivity #2	
	SOURCE: Blood	
	SITE:	
	GRAM STAIN RESULTS	
	CULTURE RESULTS: E. coli	
	SUSCEPTIBILITY:	
9/10	AMPICILLIN	R
	CEFAZOLIN	S
	CEFOTAXIME	S
	CEFTRIAXONE	S
	CEFUROXIME	S
	CEPHALOTHIN	S
	CIPROFLOXACIN	S
	ERYTHROMYCIN	S
	GENTAMICIN	S
	OXACILLIN	S
	PENICILLIN	R
	PIPERACILLIN	
	TETRACYCLINE	
	TOBRAMYCIN	
	TRIMETH/SULF	
	VANCOMYCIN	

S = SUSCEPTIBLE
R = RESISTANT
I = INTERMEDIATE
M = MODERATELY SUSCEP

RADIOLOGY REPORT—Patient 17

DATE: 9/8

CHEST X-RAY: The examination is of a recumbent AP view. Heart size is normal. The aorta is normal and lung fields are free of infiltration. There is no free air and the trachea is midline.

DIAGNOSIS: Normal chest x-ray

RADIOLOGY REPORT—Patient 17

DATE: 9/8

PYELOGRAM: The urinary architecture is normal with no hydronephrosis.

DIAGNOSIS: Normal pyelogram

PATIENT 17

ICD-9-CM CODES

PDX					.		
DX2					.		
DX3					.		
DX4					.		
DX5					.		
DX6					.		
DX7					.		
DX8					.		
DX9					.		
DX10					.		

ICD-9-CM CODES

PP1			.		
PR2			.		
PR3			.		
PR4			.		
PR5			.		
PR6			.		

INPATIENT RECORD

DISCHARGE SUMMARY—Patient 18

DATE OF ADMISSION: 9/25 **DATE OF DISCHARGE**: 9/26

DISCHARGE DIAGNOSIS:

1. Dehydration
2. Diarrhea probable due to side effect of Sinemet
3. Parkinson's disease
4. Hypertension
5. Chronic kidney disease
6. CHF

Patient is a 75-year-old woman with a history of severe Parkinson's disease admitted on 9/25 and discharged with a diagnosis of dehydration secondary to severe diarrhea.

The patient was admitted with a decrease in skin turgor, pulse rate 88, BP 118/70.

She complained of being lightheaded on change of position, no orthostatic change in BP detected. Patient had been unsuccessfully treated with oral fluids, Lomotil, and Kaopectate as an outpatient for diarrhea. Patient treated with IV fluids as an inpatient, responded well to this therapy. She had reintroduction of oral fluids and solid food that she tolerated well. The etiology of her GI complaints were thought to be due to Sinemet. Throat cultures for pathogen and bacteria were negative. CBC showed WBC 9,200 with normal differential. Hct 38.1, SMA-6 consistent with mild dehydration and CRF. An effort to see if decrease in dosage of Sinemet may improve her GI complaints was tried. We decreased her Sinemet to 3 times per day, dosage of 25 100-mg tablets.

Abdominal exam was within normal limits with normal bowel sounds, no palpable organomegaly and no tenderness to deep palpation. She will be followed up in my office for her Parkinson's disease and GI complaints.

HISTORY AND PHYSICAL EXAMINATION—Patient 18

ADMITTED: 9/25

REASON FOR ADMISSION: Dehydration, diarrhea possible secondary to side-effect of Sinemet. Parkinson's disease.

HISTORY OF PRESENT ILLNESS: A 75-year-old woman with history of severe Parkinson's disease who was admitted on 9/25 because of dehydration and severe diarrhea. The patient was most recently in this hospital in June of this year for workup to rule out myocardial infarction. Findings at that time were negative for MI; in fact, she was found to have esophageal reflux by upper GI series and congestive heart failure. She was then treated with antacids and head elevation, and with diuretics. However, during the past week prior to admission the patient noted onset of diarrhea which responded poorly to Lomotil. She continued to take Kaopectate and Lomotil p.r.n. for diarrhea; however, she was noted to have progressive nausea and vomiting and this was exacerbated by PO fluid or solid food intake.

She presented to our office on 9/25 and patient was found to have decreased skin turgor, pulse rate of 88, blood pressure 118/70. The patient complained of being lightheaded on change of position. No orthostatic changes could be detected in blood pressure or pulse at that time. The patient appeared weak. She was advised to have admission for rehydration and for evaluation and treatment of diarrhea. Patient offered no complaints of abdominal pain. There was no evidence of heartburn. Her congestive heart failure, hypertension, and chronic kidney disease are stable.

She denies alcohol use and does not smoke cigarettes.

The patient's Parkinson's disease has been fairly well controlled on Sinemet, 25 100-mg PO, q.i.d. However, this is contributing to patient's GI upset. She notes that at least once approximately one year ago she experienced similar symptoms, which cleared spontaneously with IV fluids.

For details of patient's past history, please see old chart. In summary, patient has Parkinson's disease as described above.

ALLERGIES: None known

HISTORY AND PHYSICAL EXAMINATION—Patient 18

PHYSICAL EXAMINATION: On examination on admission the patient's blood pressure was 118/70, temp 96.6, pulse 90. Decreased skin turgor noted.

HEENT: Eyes appear slightly sunken. Sclera muddy. No icterus. Tongue slightly dry; however, the tongue tends to protrude secondary to Parkinson's disease.

NECK: No neck vein distention. Neck is supple.

LUNGS: Clear

HEART: No murmur or gallop audible, positive S3.

ABDOMEN: Good bowel sounds, slightly increased. There is some deep tenderness in mid epigastric area. No rebound tenderness.

EXTREMITIES: Lower extremities—no edema or cyanosis

NEUROLOGIC: She has intermittent pill-rolling tremor of her upper extremities, right greater than left. Slightly unsteady gait on ambulation. No focal neurologic deficits.

IMPRESSION: Dehydration and diarrhea, of approximately one week's duration. Of concern is possible Sinemet side effect with gastrointestinal symptoms. Hypertension, chronic renal disease, and congestive heart failure—stable.

PLAN: Will decrease dosage of Sinemet to three tablets per day, hydrate the patient with IV fluids, treat the nausea p.r.n. with Tigan suppositories. Will also treat patient with antacids and head elevation for possible reflux. Hold dig, diuretic and ACE for now. Hold Calan SR 120 mg PO b.i.d.

Further orders per patient's course.

PROGRESS NOTES—Patient 18

DATE	NOTES
09/25	Attending MD: The patient is admitted with decreased skin turgor, secondary to dehydration caused by diarrhea. R/O side effect of Sinemet. Continue with PO fluids and solid food as tolerated. Hold digoxin, diuretic, and ACE for now. Hold Calan SR.
09/25	Nursing: Alert and oriented. IV running well, taking liquid diet, no diarrhea at present.
09/25	Nursing: Alert and oriented. No complaints offered at present. IV infusing as ordered.
09/25	Nursing: Patient comfortable, sleeping at this time.
09/26	Attending MD: Patient comfortable, tolerating solid foods, IV discontinued, will discharge today. Restart outpatient meds.
09/26	Nursing: Discharged via wheelchair to front door. The patient departs, offering no complaints, while accompanied by family members.

PHYSICIAN'S ORDERS—Patient 18

DATE	ORDER
09/25	Admission for dehydration, possibly due to Sinemet Clear liquids as tolerated, advance diet as tolerated IV D5 1/2 NS at 100 cc/h Hold Sinemet today Tigan suppositories p.r.n. nausea Elevate patient's head for probable esophageal reflux
09/26	Resume Sinemet 25/100 tablets t.i.d. D/C IV Discharge on: Digoxin 0.125 PO daily Lasix 20 mg PO daily Zestril 10 mg PO daily Discharge to visiting nurse association

LABORATORY REPORTS—Patient 18

HEMATOLOGY

DATE: 9/25

Specimen	Results	Normal Values
WBC	9.6	4.3–11.0
RBC	5.0	4.5–5.9
HGB	16.0	13.5–17.5
HCT	48	41–52
MCV	80	80–100
MCHC	33	31–57
PLT	300	150–400

CHEMISTRY

DATE: 9/25

Specimen	Results	Normal Values
GLUC	105	70–110
BUN	35 H	8–25
CREAT	1.8 H	0.5–1.5
NA	148 H	136–146
K	5.4	3.5–5.5
CL	106	95–110
CO2	30	24–32
CA	9.0	8.4–10.5
PHOS	2.9	2.5–4.4
MG	2.5	1.6–3.0
T BILI	1.0	0.2–1.2
D BILI	0.03	0.0–0.5
PROTEIN	6.8	6.0–8.0
ALBUMIN	5.1	5.0–5.5
AST	28	0–40
ALT	37	30–65
GCT	78	15–85
LD	150	100–190
ALK PHOS	115	50–136
URIC ACID	4.2	2.2–7.7
CHOL	146	0–200
TRIG	140	10–160

URINALYSIS

DATE: 9/25

Test	Result	Ref Range
SP GRAVITY	1.015	1.005–1.035
PH	5.8	5–7
PROT	NEG	NEG
GLUC	NEG	NEG
KETONES	NEG	NEG
BILI	NEG	NEG
BLOOD	NEG	NEG
LEU EST	NEG	NEG
NITRATES	NEG	NE
RED SUBS	NEG	NEG

PATIENT 18

	ICD-9-CM CODES						
PDX					.		
DX2					.		
DX3					.		
DX4					.		
DX5					.		
DX6					.		
DX7					.		
DX8					.		
DX9					.		
DX10					.		

	ICD-9-CM CODES				
PP1			.		
PR2			.		
PR3			.		
PR4			.		
PR5			.		
PR6			.		

INPATIENT RECORD

DEATH DISCHARGE SUMMARY—Patient 19

DATE OF ADMISSION: 6/22 **DATE OF DISCHARGE**: 6/25

DISCHARGE DIAGNOSIS:

1. Idiopathic thrombocytopenic purpura
2. Chronic alcoholism
3. Type I diabetes mellitus
4. Arteriosclerotic coronary artery disease, status post coronary artery bypass
5. Hyperlipidemia
6. Hypertension

ADMISSION HISTORY: This is the second admission for this 74-year-old white male with a history of type I diabetes mellitus, chronic coronary artery disease, status post coronary artery bypass, chronic hyperlipidemia, and chronic hypertension. The patient was found to have a low platelet count two weeks ago. This was originally thought to be due to a drug reaction. However, a subsequent course showed it to be probably ITP. He was initially hospitalized and given intravenous platelets and prednisone with the rise of this platelet count to over 70,000. It had been as low as 9,000. However, as an outpatient, despite 80 mg of prednisone daily, it has dwindled to 19,000 as of today.

His previous bone marrow study just showed plenty of megacaryocytes with probable peripheral destruction. There was a question of iron deficiency anemia.

COURSE IN HOSPITAL: The patient was admitted for treatment of ITP. Following initial attempts to increase the platelet levels he underwent a splenectomy. Postoperatively he experienced respiratory distress. Although platelet levels increased, his overall health deteriorated. He was pronounced dead on 6/25.

HISTORY AND PHYSICAL EXAMINATION—Patient 19

ADMITTED: 6/22

REASON FOR ADMISSION: Idiopathic thrombocytopenic purpura

HISTORY OF PRESENT ILLNESS: This is the second admission for this 74-year-old white male with a history of type I diabetes mellitus, chronic coronary artery disease, status post coronary artery bypass, chronic hyperlipidemia, and chronic hypertension. The patient was found to have a low platelet count two weeks ago. This was originally thought to be due to a drug reaction. However, a subsequent course showed it to be probably ITP. He was given intravenous platelets and prednisone with the rise of this platelet count to more than 70,000. It had been as low as 9,000. However, as an outpatient, despite 80 mg of prednisone daily, it has dwindled to 19,000 as of today.

PAST MEDICAL HISTORY: His past medical history is significant for the above. He denies recent angina spells. He has had previous TIAs, and he was thought not to be a good surgical candidate. A previous CT scan of the brain was normal.

ALLERGIES: He has no known drug allergies.

CHRONIC MEDICATIONS: Humulin 70/30 24 units b.i.d., Tenormin 25 mg PO q.d.

SOCIAL HISTORY: He stopped his previous heavy alcohol intake approximately one month ago.

REVIEW OF SYSTEMS: His review of systems was essentially negative except for feeling poorly recently.

PHYSICAL EXAMINATION:

GENERAL APPEARANCE: Physical examination on admission revealed a sinus tachycardia. Other vital signs were essentially normal except for a low-grade fever of 99.9. Respiratory rate was 28.

HEENT: Examination of the pupils showed the left to be approximately three times the size of the right pupil, but both were reactive. There was normal extraocular movement.

NECK: There was no jugular venous distention.

LUNGS: Clear to auscultation and percussion.

HEART: Cardiac examination revealed a loud S1 and sinus tachycardia.

ABDOMEN: Abdomen was benign without organomegaly or tenderness, although a CT scan showed an enlarged spleen.

EXTREMITIES: Extremities showed purpura without edema.

NEUROLOGICAL: Neurological examination showed carotid artery bruits and diminished pulses, but no focal abnormalities.

IMPRESSION:

1. Thrombocytopenia, probably idiopathic thrombocytopenic purpura
2. Chronic hypertension
3. Type 1 diabetes mellitus
4. Status post coronary bypass surgery

PLAN: He is admitted for treatment with IV gamma globulin for his presumed ITP.

PROGRESS NOTES—Patient 19

DATE	NOTE
6/22	Attending Physician: The patient is admitted for evaluation and treatment of ITP. This is a 74-year-old male in stable health. He is alert and oriented. He is a former heavy drinker. Treatment with platelets and steroids.
6/23	Attending Physician: Platelet count continues to decrease. Will consult surgery for possible splenectomy. Surgical Consult: Patient examined. The risks and benefits of surgery explained and discussed. Patient is agreeable to surgery tomorrow morning.
6/24	Surgeon's Note: Preop Dx: ITP Postop Dx: Same plus cirrhosis of the liver due to alcohol use Procedure: Splenectomy Anes: GET Patient developed respiratory distress following extubation in the recovery room. Currently in ICU. Ventilator managed by anesthesia. Anesthesia: The patient currently in ICU developed very rapid shallow breathing postop and became combative. The patient was given Valium and he began to calm. The patient has decreased urinary output. Will increase IV to 125 cc/hr. Anesthesia: The patient is currently breathing on his own via endotracheal tube. Will return in p.m. to extubate the patient. Attending Note: The patient is now extubated and resting comfortably. Continue to monitor.
6/25	House Physician: Called to the floor to examine this 74-year-old male, postop one day. He was found unresponsive on the floor. There were no pulses or respirations. Code called, however, was unsuccessful. The patient was pronounced at 4:45 a.m. Attending Physician: The patient's course discussed with the patient's family. Condolences expressed.

PHYSICIAN'S ORDERS—Patient 19

DATE	ORDER
6/22	Attending MD: Patient admitted for treatment of ITP 2 units of platelets Gamma globulin Type and cross 2 units PRBCs Tenormin 25 mg q.d Prednisone 40 mg b.i.d. Humulin 70/30 24 units b.i.d VS q. 3 hours BS q. 2 hours
6/23	Attending MD: Consult Surgery re: Splenectomy Surgery: NPO after 6 p.m. FBS done before OR Valium 20 mg in a.m. Decrease insulin to 12 units for evening and preop dose
6/24	Surgery: Admit to ICU Postop respiratory distress Vent settings as per anesthesia ½ NSS 80 cc/hr Transfuse 2 units PRBCs Daily FBS Anesthesia: Transfer patient to floor
6/25	Release body to coroner

OPERATIVE REPORT—Patient 19

DATE: 6/24

PREOPERATIVE DIAGNOSIS: Idiopathic thrombocytopenic purpura

POSTOPERATIVE DIAGNOSIS: Same

OPERATION: Splenectomy

ANESTHESIA: General endotracheal

OPERATIVE INDICATIONS: Uncontrolled decreasing platelets

OPERATIVE PROCEDURE: The patient was brought to the operating room where he was placed in the supine position and prepped and draped in the usual manner. Following the induction of anesthesia, an incision was made. The abdominal cavity was entered. The liver was also found to be cirrhotic. A splenectomy was performed and the patient closed.

The patient tolerated the procedure well and was sent to the recovery room in stable condition.

PATHOLOGY REPORT—Patient 19

DATE: 6/24

SPECIMEN: Spleen

CLINICAL DATA: 74-year-old male with ITP

DIAGNOSIS: Spleen with increased megacaryocytes indicative of ITP

LABORATORY REPORTS—Patient 19

HEMATOLOGY

DATE: 6/22

Specimen	Results	Normal Values
WBC	5.0	4.3–11.0
RBC	4.3 L	4.5–5.9
HGB	12.5 L	13.5–17.5
HCT	39 L	41–52
MCV	91	80–100
MCHC	47	31–57
PLT	19 L	150–400

DATE: 6/23

Specimen	Results	Normal Values
WBC	5.0	4.3–11.0
RBC	4.3 L	4.5–5.9
HGB	12.5 L	13.5–17.5
HCT	39 L	41–52
MCV	91	80–100
MCHC	47	31–57
PLT	17 L	150–400

DATE: 6/24

Specimen	Results	Normal Values
WBC	5.0	4.3–11.0
RBC	4.0 L	4.5–5.9
HGB	11.6 L	13.5–17.5
HCT	35 L	41–52
MCV	91	80–100
MCHC	47	31–57
PLT	19 L	150–400

CHEMISTRY—Patient 19

Specimen	Results			Normal Values
	6/22	6/23	6/24	
GLUC	115 H	118 H	125 H	70–110
BUN	20	18	27 H	8–25
CREAT	1.0	1.0	1.0	0.5–1.5
NA	138	140	130L	136–146
K	4.0	4.5	5.4	3.5–5.5
CL	100			95–110
CO2	30			24–32
CA	9.0			8.4–10.5
PHOS	3.0			2.5–4.4
MG				1.6–3.0
T BILI				0.2–1.2
D BILI				0.0–0.5
PROTEIN				6.0–8.0
ALBUMIN				5.0–5.5
AST	65 H	64 H	65H	0–40
ALT	79 H	82 H	77H	30–65
GCT				15–85
LD				100–190
ALK PHOS				50–136
URIC ACID				2.2–7.7
CHOL				0–200
TRIG				10–160

RADIOLOGY REPORT—Patient 19

DATE: 6/22

DIAGNOSIS: ITP

EXAMINATION: Chest x-ray

Heart size and shape are acceptable. The lung fields are clear and the pulmonary vascular pattern is unremarkable. There is no free fluid and the trachea remains midline.

IMPRESSION: Unremarkable chest x-ray

PATIENT 19

ICD-9-CM CODES

					.		
PDX					.		
DX2					.		
DX3					.		
DX4					.		
DX5					.		
DX6					.		
DX7					.		
DX8					.		
DX9					.		
DX10					.		

ICD-9-CM CODES

PP1			.		
PR2			.		
PR3			.		
PR4			.		
PR5			.		
PR6			.		

INPATIENT RECORD

DISCHARGE SUMMARY—Patient 20

DATE OF ADMISSION: 1/27 **DATE OF DISCHARGE**: 1/29

DISCHARGE DIAGNOSIS: Nonrheumatic congestive heart failure

ADMISSION HISTORY: This is a 57-year-old married white gentleman, referred because of recurrent shortness of breath and cough. He states that he was in his usual state of good health until approximately Christmas, when he developed a persistent cough with associated dyspnea. His dyspnea was most prominent with exertion. He was treated with Ceclor at that time, with some improvement. However, his symptoms recurred and he underwent a second course of antibiotics, again with some improvement. However, his symptoms have now recurred and he is referred for further evaluation.

He has known tricuspid insufficiency, mild left ventricular dysfunction and left ventricular dilatation by echocardiogram done 6/2. He had a normal stress ECG 10/3. The patient also has hypertension.

COURSE IN HOSPITAL: The patient was referred because of recurrent shortness of breath and cough. Apparently the patient had been doing well up until Christmas. His cough was treated with antibiotics with some improvement. His symptoms, however, recurred, requiring a second course of antibiotics.

The patient was admitted with a diagnosis of congestive heart failure. He was started on diuretics with improvement in his physical examination and his symptoms. An echocardiogram was performed, which is described as above.

The patient was extremely anxious to go home and thought that the rest of his care could be accomplished as an outpatient. He is tolerating his medications and will remain on the Capoten and the Lasix and will have a follow-up appointment with his doctor in one to two weeks and I will see him again in approximately four weeks. It is recommended at that time that discussion for cardiac catheterization be carried out. This was discussed with the patient during his hospitalization, the reason being that perhaps his aortic insufficiency is more significant than what is appreciated on physical examination and by echocardiogram. The catheterization would aid in the evaluation of the etiology of his LV dysfunction and his left ventricular enlargement. He has also been given information about smoking cessation.

INSTRUCTIONS ON DISCHARGE: 1. Capoten 12.5 mg b.i.d., 2. Lasix 40 mg daily; 3. Insulin Humulin N 14 in a.m. with 6 of regular and Humulin N 20 units in the p.m. with 12 of regular.

HISTORY AND PHYSICAL EXAMINATION—Patient 20

ADMITTED: 1/27

REASON FOR ADMISSION: This is a 57-year-old married white gentleman, referred because of recurrent shortness of breath and cough. He states that he was in his usual state of good health until approximately Christmas, when he developed a persistent cough with associated dyspnea. His dyspnea was most prominent with exertion. He was treated with Ceclor at that time with some improvement. However, his symptoms recurred and he underwent a second course of antibiotics, again with some improvement. However, his symptoms have now recurred and he is referred for further evaluation.

He has known moderate tricuspid valve insufficiency, mild left ventricular dysfunction and left ventricular dilatation by echocardiogram. He had a normal stress ECG on 10/3.

PAST MEDICAL HISTORY: The patient has a history of type I diabetes mellitus. He believes that his most recent cholesterol reading was under 200. He previously has been hospitalized for pericarditis and for resection of popliteal artery aneurysm. He has a history of hypertension.

ALLERGIES: None known

CHRONIC MEDICATIONS: Humulin Insulin 6 units of R and 14 units of N in the morning and 12 units of R and 20 units of N in the evening. Lotensin 20 mg PO daily.

He denies any drug allergies.

FAMILY HISTORY: Noncontributory

SOCIAL HISTORY: The patient is married and lives with his wife and smokes one to two packs of cigarettes per day.

REVIEW OF SYSTEMS: Otherwise noncontributory

HISTORY AND PHYSICAL EXAMINATION—Patient 20

PHYSICAL EXAMINATION: Reveals a blood pressure of 140/80, pulse 80 and regular. The patient was a pleasant, adult, white male who is in no acute distress. His carotids were without bruits. The jugular venous pulse was normal. Examination of his lungs was remarkable for fine, bibasilar rales. On auscultation of his heart, he has a regular rhythm, a soft murmur consistent with tricuspid insuffiency. Abdominal examination was unremarkable except for the presence of a liver edge just below the costal margin. He had no peripheral edema.

LABORATORY DATA: Thyroid function tests were within normal limits. Total cholesterol level was 194. His HDL and LDL are presently still pending. His blood sugar levels have been well controlled in the low 100s. His electrolytes and SMA 12 are normal as well as his complete blood count.

His EKG on admission revealed sinus rhythm with left atrial enlargement, nonspecific ST-T wave abnormality with poor R wave progression, no acute changes.

His echocardiogram revealed left ventricular enlargement, normal left atrial size at 4 cm, mild overall reduction of left ventricular contractility with diffuse hypokinesis, mild to moderate tricuspid insufficiency.

IMPRESSION:

1. Persistent shortness of breath and cough—possible nonrheumatic congestive heart failure; rule out persistent respiratory tract infection
2. Tricuspid insufficiency, left ventricular dysfunction/dilatation, by echocardiogram
3. Type I diabetes mellitus
4. Smoking history

CONSULTATION—Patient 20

DATE: 1/28

Podiatric consultation was requested. The patient's chart was reviewed in the following manner: H & P, Labs, progress notes, physician's orders, previous consultations and any other pertinent information remaining in the patient's chart.

CHIEF COMPLAINT: Diabetic foot care

PHYSICAL EXAMINATION: The patient is a 57-year-old white male admitted with a history of hypertension and diabetes mellitus, insulin dependent for approximately seven years. The patient has shortness of breath and is a smoker. The patient states that he has had a problem with one of the valves in his heart for approximately three years. The patient had resection of an aneurysm in the right leg in 1989. The patient has no known drug allergies. Multiple nails, right and left feet are hypertrophic and mycotic with in-growing tendencies. The patient has had trauma to both the great toenails at the age of 12 years due to a vehicular accident. Gait analysis will be deferred at this time. Pulses are present in both feet and ankles. The toes are warm. There are no digital lesions at this time. The muscle tone and power are fair. The patient denied having intermittent claudication during gait or phlebitis affecting either lower extremity. The patient does have some numbness of the right great toe, status post surgery for the popliteal aneurysm.

IMPRESSION:

Type I diabetes mellitus
Congestive heart failure
Valvular heart disease
Smoker
Status post resection of aneurysm of the right leg
Hypertension

PLAN: Podiatric consultation; initial; comprehensive. Debridement of hypertrophic mycotic nail plates bilateral feet—symptomatic.

PROCEDURE: Debridement of hypertrophic mycotic nail plates, bilateral feet, symptomatic

RECOMMENDATIONS: Diabetic foot care q. 1 to 3 months. The patient will be followed p.r.n.

PROGRESS NOTES—Patient 20

DATE	NOTE
1/27	Physical examination reveals rales and evidence of valvular heart disease. Will diurese with Lasix and obtain an echocardiogram.
1/28	Patient better today—no shortness of breath, no edema. The importance of smoking cessation was discussed with the patient.
1/29	Will discharge the patient today.

PHYSICIAN'S ORDERS—Patient 20

DATE	ORDER
1/27	Chest x-ray Monitor input and output Lasix 40 mg IV now and 40 mg PO in a.m. Schedule patient for an echocardiogram CBC Consult podiatry for diabetic foot care Lotensin 20 mg PO daily in a.m.
1/23	Discharge patient to home

LABORATORY REPORTS—Patient 20

HEMATOLOGY

DATE: 1/27

Specimen	Results	Normal Values
WBC	10	4.3–11.0
RBC	5.0	4.5–5.9
HGB	16.2	13.5–17.5
HCT	48	41–52
MCV	93	80–100
MCHC	35	31–57
PLT	339	150–400

RADIOLOGY REPORT—Patient 20

DATE: 1/28

Chest x-ray

DIAGNOSIS: The examination is compared to a prior examination on March 2 of last year. The cardiac silhouette remains at the upper limits of normal in size. The pulmonary vascularity appears slightly congested and there is a right-sided pleural effusion that was not present on the prior examination. There is minimal blunting of the left costophrenic angle. The appearance suggests congestive heart failure.

IMPRESSION: Findings of congestive heart failure

PATIENT 20

ICD-9-CM CODES

PDX					.		
DX2					.		
DX3					.		
DX4					.		
DX5					.		
DX6					.		
DX7					.		
DX8					.		
DX9					.		
DX10					.		

ICD-9-CM CODES

PP1			.		
PR2			.		
PR3			.		
PR4			.		
PR5			.		
PR6			.		

INPATIENT RECORD

DISCHARGE SUMMARY—Patient 21

DATE OF ADMISSION: 10/21 **DATE OF DISCHARGE**: 10/22

DISCHARGE DIAGNOSIS: Retained products of conception with vaginal bleeding following dilation and curettage (D & C) for miscarriage and tobacco and alcohol abuse.

COURSE IN HOSPITAL: The patient was admitted to the emergency department due to fainting and vaginal bleeding. The patient was taken to the OR for D & C. Pathology revealed desidua and chronic villa. She previously underwent a D & C for a miscarriage last week at another institution. The patient was encouraged to decrease her alcohol intake and to stop smoking. The patient appeared depressed over her recent miscarriage. A psych consult was ordered.

INSTRUCTIONS ON DISCHARGE: If heavy bleeding occurs, contact my office immediately. A follow-up visit is scheduled for follow-up with the psychiatrist in 2 weeks. The patient was also given information about Alcoholics Anonymous as well as a prescription for Wellbutrin to be taken as directed for depression and smoking cessation.

HISTORY AND PHYSICAL EXAMINATION—Patient 21

ADMITTED: 10/21

REASON FOR ADMISSION: Heavy bleeding from vagina

HISTORY OF PRESENT ILLNESS: She has had irregular spotting and light flow on and off since a spontaneous abortion that occurred last week. She was admitted to another hospital at that time and underwent a D & C. The patient noted heavy bleeding today. She fainted in the bathroom and was brought to the emergency department by her family.

PAST MEDICAL HISTORY: The patient developed bronchitis as a child, but was not treated other than with decongestant. Her last menstrual period was 6 weeks ago.

ALLERGIES: None known

CHRONIC MEDICATIONS: None

FAMILY HISTORY: Mother has hypertension. Two sisters have had heart surgery for congenital heart problems.

SOCIAL HISTORY: The patient smokes one pack of cigarettes per day and reports intake of one six-pack every few days during the week. The patient tried to abstain from alcohol during her pregnancy but was not successful.

REVIEW OF SYSTEMS: The patient is normally healthy. She has had a runny nose for about two days. Her bowel movements are normal, once every 2 to 3 days and her urinary function is normal. She eats three meals per day. She gets heartburn when she eats spicy foods. She drinks with her meals and into the evening on a continual basis.

PHYSICAL EXAMINATION:

HEENT: PERRL, EOM normal, thyroid not enlarged

CHEST: Clear to P & A without CVA tenderness

HEART: NSR without murmur

ABDOMEN: Soft and nontender with active bowel sounds

EXTREMITIES: Without edema, cyanosis, or clubbing

NEURO: CN's II–XII grossly intact. Reflexes are normal. No sensory or motor defects noted.

PELVIC: Uterus is of normal size with AV and femoral adnexa negative. Vaginal vault filled with serum fluid and clots. Cervix reveals pink with blood oozing from OS—no foreign body or laceration noted.

ASSESSMENT: Dysfunctional uterine bleeding

PLAN: D & C

CONSULTATION—Patient 21

Psych Consult

Thank you for requesting a consult with this patient. I met with her and found her to be depressed secondary to recent miscarriage. There was no evidence of suicidal thoughts. She denies any thoughts of harming herself or others. The patient has a history of alcohol abuse, three 6-packs of beer per week, and tobacco 1 ppd.

IMPRESSION:

1. Depression—secondary to recent miscarriage
2. Alcohol abuse
3. Tobacco abuse

Will treat with Wellbutrin 150 mg PO daily × 3 days then BID thereafter. F/U in 2 weeks.

PROGRESS NOTES—Patient 21

DATE	NOTE
10/21	The patient has been bleeding for approximately 1 week utilizing at least 3 pads per day for flow of blood. We will repeat the D & C to determine if the patient has retained products of conception. **PREOPERATIVE DIAGNOSIS**: Severe menorrhagia **POSTOPERATIVE DIAGNOSIS**: Same **OPERATION**: Dilatation and curettage **ANESTHESIA**: Paracervical block using 1% Xylocaine and sedation using IV Valium The patient tolerated the procedure well. Await pathology report. The patient appears depressed, will order a psych consult.
10/22	The patient has decreased bleeding with decreased cramping. Will discharge today. Psych consult appreciated. The importance of decreasing alcohol and tobacco use was stressed as was the effect of these substances on fetal development. The patient will follow up with the psychiatrist after discharge.

PHYSICIAN'S ORDERS—Patient 21

DATE	ORDER
10/21	Admit the patient to the labor and delivery floor Vaginal prep 1,000 cc LR NPO Type and screen CBC Psych consult
10/22	Discharge patient to home

OPERATIVE REPORT—Patient 21

DATE: 10/21

PREOPERATIVE DIAGNOSIS: Severe menorrhagia

POSTOPERATIVE DIAGNOSIS: Same

OPERATION: Dilatation and curettage

ANESTHESIA: Paracervical block using 1% Xylocaine and sedation using IV Valium

OPERATIVE PROCEDURE: The patient was brought to the operating room and placed in the supine position. After IV Valium sedation, the patient was placed in the lithotomy position. The vaginal and perineal areas were then prepped and draped in the usual manner for vaginal surgery. Weighted speculum was inserted and the anterior retractor was used to expose the cervix. The cervix was then grasped using the Jacob's tenaculum. The paracervical block was then performed and then using Pratt dilators, the cervix was dilated up to #23. The uterus was then sounded and found to be approximately 7.5 cm. Using a medium sized sharp curette, the uterine cavity was then curetted in systematic fashion from twelve o'clock clockwise to six o'clock and then from twelve o'clock counterclockwise to six o'clock. Endometrial tissue obtained was sent to pathology. The Jacob's tenaculum was removed and with assurance of hemostasis, the weighted speculum was removed. The patient tolerated the procedure and anesthesia well and arrived in the recovery room in satisfactory condition.

PATHOLOGY REPORT—Patient 21

DATE: 10/22

GROSS DESCRIPTION: Labeled "endometrium" are multiple irregular fragments of tan-white tissue and blood clots, forming a spheroid 1.0 cm in diameter. All blocked.

MICROSCOPIC DESCRIPTION:

DIAGNOSIS: Secretory endometrium, with necrotic fragments of decidua and chorionic villi, consistent with retained products of conception

LABORATORY REPORTS—Patient 21

HEMATOLOGY

DATE: 10/21

Specimen	Results	Normal Values
WBC	10	4.3–11.0
RBC	5.0	4.5–5.9
HGB	13.5	13.5–17.5
HCT	41	41–52
MCV	93	80–100
MCHC	35	31–57
PLT	339	150–400

PATIENT 21

ICD-9-CM CODES

PDX					.		
DX2					.		
DX3					.		
DX4					.		
DX5					.		
DX6					.		
DX7					.		
DX8					.		
DX9					.		
DX10					.		

ICD-9-CM CODES

PP1			.		
PR2			.		
PR3			.		
PR4			.		
PR5			.		
PR6			.		

Congratulations! You have completed the 13 patient records!

To continue your steps to success

- Identify any areas that need improvement
- Research and reviewing study resources for clarification
- Seek assistance from CCS-credentialed professionals
- Practice, practice, practice

Good luck on the examination!

Coding Practice Answer Key

Answers for ICD-9-CM Coding Practice

Infectious and Parasitic Diseases

1. 042; 482.40
2. 550.90; 042; 53.02
3. 599.0; 041.4

Endocrine, Nutritional, and Metabolic Diseases and Immunity Disorders

1. 250.80; 707.14
2. 244.0
3. 276.51; 438.82; 787.20

Mental Disorders

1. 296.80
2. 296.24
3. 303.00; 571.2; 305.40; 94.68

Diseases of the Blood and Blood Forming Organs, Nervous System and Sense Organs

1. 280.0; 531.40
2. 345.9; 350.1; (*Coding Clinic* 1st Quarter, 2008)
3. 366.17; 250.00; 401.9; 584.9
4. 434.91; 784.3; 342.90

Diseases of the Respiratory System

1. 486; 427.31. In accordance with the UHDDS, both conditions are not equally treated. The pneumonia was treated with IV antibiotics. This diagnosis had greater utilization of resources of medications and staff time compared with the atrial fibrillation, which was treated with oral medication. Because of this, the pneumonia is sequenced first.
2. 491.21; 403.91, 585.5
3. 518.81, 428.0; 401.9

Diseases of the Digestive System

1. 571.5; 456.20
2. 560.81; 54.59
3. 574.10; 575.8; V64.41; 51.22, 54.59
4. V76.51, 211.3;V16.0; 45.42 (*Coding Clinic* 4th Quarter 2001, 11–12)

Diseases of the Genitourinary System

1. 592.0; 591; 56.0
2. 618.09; 70.51

Diseases of Skin and Subcutaneous Tissue

1. 707.07; 715.36; 86.22
2. 682.6; 989.5
3. 706.2; 86.3
4. 172.5; 86.4

Diseases of the Musculoskeletal System and Connective Tissue

1. 722.10; 80.51
2. 733.13; 733.00

Complications of Pregnancy and Childbirth Complications, Abortion, Congenital Anomalies, and Perinatal Conditions

1. 663.31; V27.0; 73.6
2. 656.61; 666.02; V27.0; 72.1
3. 651.01; 644.21; 73.59; V27.2
4. 650; V27.0; 73.6
5. 633.10; 66.62

6. 634.91; 69.52. This represents an incomplete spontaneous abortion as evidenced by the vaginal bleeding. The D & C is the method used to complete the miscarriage.
7. 639.3
8. 745.5
9. V30.01; 767.8
10. V30.00; 765.28
11. V32.01; 765.14; 773.1, 765.26

Disease of the Circulatory System

1. 414.01; 411.1; 37.21. The clinical scenario is one typical of unstable angina. (*Coding Clinic* 3rd Quarter 1990, 6–10). The coronary artery disease is coded as principal. (*Coding Clinic* 2rd Quarter 2004, 3)
2. 428.0
3. 428.0; 401.9
4. 584.9; 401.9

Neoplasms

1. 162.5; 198.3; 32.49
2. 174.2; 196.3; 85.21: 40.3
3. 185; 197.7; 62.41
4. 276.51; 197.6; 183.0, 789.51 (*Coding Clinic* 2rd Quarter 2007, 95–96)
5. 162.5; 33.27
6. 188.8; 57.49
7. 198.5; 199.1
8. 173.7
9. 197.7; V10.3, V45.71
10. 162.9; 199.1

Injuries

1. 921.3
2. 801.00
3. 800.12
4. 836.1
5. 823.31; 822.0; 79.26

Burns

1. 945.26
2. 942.33; 948.21

Poisoning and Adverse Effects of Drugs

1. 969.4; 963.0; 780.2; E853.2*; E858.1*. The patient took over-the-counter medications with a prescription medication without consulting the prescribing physician. This is a poisoning. (Refer to *Coding Clinic* 2nd Quarter 2002 and *ICD-9-CM Official Coding Guidelines*.)
2. 451.19; 964.2; 965.1; 782.7; 724.5; E858.2*; E850.3*
3. 965.09; E950.0*
4. 995.20; E933.0*

Complications of Surgical and Medical Care

1. 996.42, V43.64
2. 996.72
3. 997.02; 434.91. Categories in 997 require a second code as per the instructions under the main heading in the tabular index.
4. 518.4
5. 996.64; 038.11, 995.91
6. 996.83

*For the purposes of this examination, only E-codes associated with adverse effects of drugs are coded.

Answers for CPT Coding Practice

Anesthesia

Anesthesia code for the following procedures:

1. Removal of cataract: 00142–P2 (See the Anesthesia Guidelines.)
2. Tracheotomy in 3-month-old: 00326
3. Radical mastectomy: 00404
4. Insertion central venous pressure (CVP) for venous access catheter: 00532
5. Lumbar sympathectomy: 00632
6. EGD: 00740
7. Menisectomy of the knee: 01400–P3 (See the Anesthesia Guidelines.)
8. Open reduction fracture of the distal ulna: 01830
9. Cardiac catheterization: 01920
10. Vaginal delivery: 01960

Medicine

1. Tetanus immunoglobulin IM: 90389
2. Vaccination for hepatitis A and hepatitis B, adult, IM: 90636
3. Chemotherapy for 3 hours infusion: 96413, 96415, 96415
4. Esophageal acid reflux test: 91034
5. Right and left cardiac catheterization with angiography and ventriculography: 93526, 93543, 93545, 93542, 93555, 93556

Radiology

1. Chest x-ray, two views: 71020
2. Chest x-ray, complete: 71030
3. Abdominal ultrasound: 76700
4. Mammogram of right breast: 77055–RT
5. Screening mammogram: 77057
6. Ultrasound guidance for breast needle localization placement: 77032
7. CT scan guidance for liver biopsy: 77012
8. Ultrasound of kidneys: 76770
9. CT scan of head with contrast: 70460
10. MRI of chest without contrast: 71550

Surgery—Integumentary

1. Wide excision of 0.65-cm melanoma from right forearm: 11601
2. Excision of two (2) left breast lesions: 19120–LT
3. Excision of basal cell carcinoma, 1.9 cm lesion left upper eyelid: 11642–E1
4. Removal of two (2) skin tags on chest (0.3 cm and 0.5 cm): 11200
5. Repair of laceration of left thigh (5.1 cm) with suture of epidermis and dermis: 12002
6. Repair of two (2) wounds of the neck (2.0 cm and 1.4 cm) with layered closure: 12042

Surgery—Musculoskeletal

1. Surgical arthroscopy of the left shoulder with decompression and acromioplasty: 29826–LT
2. Closed reduction of fracture of right proximal ulna: 24675–RT
3. Hallux valgus repair with resection of the joint with implant in the first left toe proximal phalanx: 28293–TA (See *CPT Assistant* Dec. 1996, 6.)
4. Open reduction with internal fixation of right humeral condylar lateral fracture: 24579–RT
5. Diagnostic arthroscopy of left knee with medial and lateral meniscus repair: 29883–LT
6. Removal of pins and screws from right ankle following open reduction and internal fixation occurring one year ago: 20680–RT
7. Posterior fasciotomy for compartment syndrome of left upper leg following recent trauma: 27496–LT

Surgery—Respiratory

1. Extensive excision of bilateral nasal polyps: 30115–50
2. Endoscopic sinusotomy with bilateral anterior ethmoidectomy: 31254–50 (*CPT Assistant* Jan. 1997, 4; Sept. 1997, 10; Oct. 1997, 5; Dec. 2001, 6; May 2003, 5)
3. Bronchoscopy with bilateral transbronchial biopsy: 31628–50 (*CPT Assistant* June 2001) Note the biopsy was not done in a different lobe of the same lung therefore 31628 and 31632 are not used.
4. Thoracoscopic pleurodesis: 32650
5. Indirect laryngoscopic removal of foreign body: 31511
6. Thoracoscopic left thoracic sympathectomy: 32664–LT
7. Percutaneous biopsy of the right lung: 32405–RT

Surgery—Cardiovascular/Lymph

1. Percutaneous balloon angioplasty of renal artery: 35471
2. Diagnostic left and right retrograde heart catheterization through left heart cath, left ventriculogram, coronary arteriogram: 93526; 93543; 93545
3. Replacement of dual chamber pacemaker generator with removal of old generator: 33213; 33233
4. Creation of arteriovenous anastomosis for renal dialysis, open; by basilic vein transposition: 36819

Surgery—Digestive

1. Rubber band hemorrhoidectomy of external hemorrhoids: 46221
2. Esophagogastroduodenoscopy with sclerotherapy of esophageal varices: 43243
3. Esophagogastroduodenoscopy with insertion of percutaneous endoscopic gastrostomy: 43246
4. Colonoscopy with cauterization of diverticular bleeding: 45382
5. Sigmoidoscopy with snare removal of polyp: 45338
6. Laparoscopic recurrent left inguinal hernia repair: 49651–LT
7. A 3-year-old male undergoes repair of an initial incarcerated right inguinal hernia: 49501–RT

Surgery—Genitourinary

1. Cystourethroscopy with removal of 1.5-cm bladder tumor: 52234
2. Cystourethroscopy with removal of ureteral calculus: 52320
3. Cystoscopy with insertion of double-J ureteral stent in right ureter: 52332–RT
4. Transurethral resection of the prostate with electrocautery: 52601
5. Laparoscopic sling procedure for urinary incontinence: 51992
6. Circumcision of 32-year-old male using clamp: 54150
7. Cryosurgical destruction of papilloma of the penis: 54056
8. Endoscopic laser destruction of endometriosis of ovary and cul-de-sac: 58662
9. Laparoscopic tubal ligation: 58670
10. Ovarian cystectomy: 58925
11. Hysteroscopy with endometrial ablation: 58563
12. Laparoscopic salpingectomy for removal of ectopic pregnancy: 59151
13. Dilatation and curettage for missed abortion at 11 weeks' gestation: 59820
14. Removal of cervical cerclage under spinal anesthesia in a pregnant woman: 59871

Surgery—Nervous

1. Blood patch for postspinal headache: 62273
2. Bilateral epidural lumbar injection of steroids: 62311; 62311

Surgery—Ocular/Auditory

1. Repair of oval window fistula: 69666
2. Extraction of extracapsular cataract with simultaneous intraocular lens insertion in the right eye: 66984–RT
3. Endolaser photocoagulation repair of retinal detachment in the left eye: 67105–LT

Answers for Emergency Room Record

1. Diagnosis: 786.59, 305.1
2. CPT code using Map 1—no meds given (5 points), history is PF (10 points), examination is EPF (15), tests are 5 (15 points), and supplies are none (points equal 0). The total points are 45. There were both radiology and lab tests done, the CPT is 99283–25.

Answers for the Sample Multiple Choice Questions

1. C
2. B
3. D
4. A
5. B
6. C 038.9 with 86.22 results in MS-DRG 855 wt. = 1.814 (D is not correct because 038.9 with 96.71 results in MS-DRG 872 wt. = 1.1209.)
7. C
8. C (*CPT Assistant* Dec. 2007, 7)
9. A
10. B
11. C
12. B

Answers for Sample Inpatient Case

PATIENT X

ICD-9-CM CODES

PDX Endometrial carcinoma		1	8	2	.	0	
DX2 Accidental laceration		9	9	8	.	2	
DX3 Post-op shock		9	9	8	.	0	
DX4 Acute blood loss anemia		2	8	5	.	1	
DX5 Chronic blood loss anemia		2	8	0	.	0	
DX6 Post-surgical hypothyroidism		2	4	4	.	0	
DX7 Intra-operative hemorrhage		9	9	8	.	1	1
DX8 Hemoperitoneum		5	6	8	.	8	1
DX9 Family history of colon cancer		V	1	6	.	0	
DX10					.		

ICD-9-CM CODES

PP1 Laparoscopic assisted vaginal hysterectomy	6	8	.	5	1
PR2 Suture of lacerated epigastric artery	3	9	.	3	1
PR3			.		
PR4			.		
PR5			.		
PR6			.		

Notes for Sample Inpatient Case

182.0 Endometrial carcinoma is documented in the pathology report and the discharge summary.

998.2 Accidental laceration is documented in the second operative report.

998.0 Postoperative shock is denoted in the discharge summary.

285.1 Acute blood loss anemia is documented in the progress notes and from the operative report because the patient had blood loss of 1,500 to 2,000 mL. The labs also reflect this diagnosis. (*Coding Clinic* 2nd Quarter, 1992)

280.0 The patient also had chronic blood loss anemia as documented on the H & P. (*Coding Clinic* 4th Quarter, 1993)

244.0 Postsurgical hypothyroidism is documented on the H & P report and patient received Synthroid while an inpatient.

998.11 Intraoperative hemorrhage documented in the operative report.

568.81 Coded to add further specificity.

Note: The chronic cervicitis is not coded because it is an incidental finding.

68.51 The patient underwent a laparoscopic-assisted vaginal hysterectomy (Do not code the laparoscopy because it is the operative approach.)

39.31 The patient underwent another laparoscopy for suture of the lacerated epigastric artery. (Do not code the laparoscopy because it is the operative approach.)

Answers for Sample Ambulatory Case

PATIENT X

ICD-9-CM CODES

PDX Left inguinal hernia		5	5	0	.	9	0
DX2 Lipoma of spermatic cord (as per path and operative report)		2	1	4	.	4	
DX3					.		
DX4					.		

CPT CODES

PP1 Hernia repair	4	9	5	0	5–LT
PR2 Excision lipoma spermatic cord (*CPT Assistant,* Sept., 2000)	5	5	5	2	0–59
PR3					
PR4					
PR5					
PR6					
PR7					

Exam Simulation Answer Key

Answers for Part I: Multiple Choice Questions

1. C
2. C (Davis/LaCour 2007, 156)
3. D (*CPT Assistant* April 2002, 20)
4. A (*Coding Clinic* 4th Quarter 2005)
5. C
6. A (Johns 2006, 718)
7. B (Davis/LaCour 2007, 130)
8. C
9. A (*CPT Assistant* March 2005, 1,4; Dec. 2005, 7; Jan. 2007, 31; *CPT Changes An Insider's View 2005*)
10. C DRG weights are multiplied by the number of patients and then divided by the total number of patients, 30 + 20 + 10 = 60/30 = 2.0.
11. A
12. D 038.9 with 96.72 results in MS-DRG 870 wt. 5.7258 (Note: The www.irp.com calculator appears to have an error. If the calculator on this site is used with the codes in answer D, it results in a DRG of 1.1209. Please refer to the FY 2009 DRG weights from Medicare at www.hhs.medicare.gov for the correct weight.) (C is not correct because 038.9 with 86.22 results in MS-DRG 855 wt. = 1.814.)
13. B
14. C The blood gas values of pO_2 of 58, pCO_2 of 55, pH of 7.32 reflect respiratory failure and the patient was treated in ICU with intubation and mechanical ventilation.
15. B MS-DRG 292
16. D (*CPT Assistant* Nov. 2002, 5)
17. D The DRG would be 264 with a weight of 2.484.
18. B
19. D
20. A

21. B The reason for the Cesarean section would be the principal diagnosis. In this case, the patient undergoes an emergency Cesarean section because of bleeding that is associated with placenta previa.

22. A

23. A If the spontaneous abortion was not completed on a previous admission, the diagnosis is spontaneous abortion in subsequent admissions until it has been completed.

24. A (*Coding Clinic* 3rd Quarter 2002, 24)

25. C

26. A

27. B

28. B

29. C

30. A (*CPT Assistant* Dec. 2007, 7)

31. C (AHIMA Standards of Ethical Coding)

32. C

33. D (www.herceptin.com)

34. C (*CPT Changes 2008—An Insider's View*)

35. C (*CPT Changes 2008—An Insider's View*)

36. D Older codes were used to highlight the need to know recent changes in codes.

37. C

38. C

39. D

40. B

41. C

42. A This is an example of a circumstance where the chronic condition must be verified. All secondary conditions must meet the UHDDS definitions and whether the COPD does is not clear (*Coding Clinic* 3rd Quarter 2007, 13–14).

43. C (Johns 2006, 357)

44. D A symptom followed by contrasting/comparative diagnoses, the symptom is sequenced first. All the contrasting/comparative diagnosis should be coded as additional diagnoses (*ICD-9-CM Official Coding Guidelines for Coding and Reporting,* Section II, E).

45. A

46. B (*Coding Clinic* 3rd Quarter 2002, 12)

47. B

48. A (Johns 2006, 745)

49. B

50. B (*Coding Clinic* 4th Quarter 2005, 78–79)

51. D (Davis/LaCour 2007, 111)

52. D (*CPT Assistant* Nov. 2002, 5)

53. A (John 2006, 836)

54. A

55. B

56. C

57. D

58. C (Johns 2006, 836)

59. B This may indicate congestive heart failure.

60. C

Answers for Part II: Outpatient Record (Patients 1–11)

PATIENT 1*

ICD-9-CM CODES

PDX Ductal carcinoma right breast		2	3	3	.	0	
DX2					.		
DX3					.		
DX4					.		

CPT CODES

PP1 Lumpectomy	1	9	3	0	1–RT
PR2 Sentinel axillary lymph node dissection	3	8	5	2	5–RT
PR3					
PR4					
PR5					
PR6					
PR7					

*Please note that the answer sheets for CCS Exam outpatient records require only 4 diagnoses and 7 procedures.

PATIENT 2

ICD-9-CM CODES

PDX	Chronic serous otitis media		3	8	1	.	1	0
DX2	Sinusitis NOS		4	7	3	.	9	
DX3	Adenoid hypertrophy		4	7	4	.	1	2
DX4						.		

CPT CODES

PP1	Myringotomy with insertion of tubes (bilateral)	6	9	4	3	6–50
PR2	Adenoidectomy (patient is 35)	4	2	8	3	1
PR3						
PR4						
PR5						
PR6						
PR7						

PATIENT 3

ICD-9-CM CODES

PDX Aphakic bullous keratopathy		3	7	1	.	2	3
DX2 Apkakia		3	7	9	.	3	1
DX3 Open-angle glaucoma		3	6	5	.	1	0
DX4 Chronic Iritis		3	6	4	.	1	0
DX5 Angina		4	1	3		9	
DX6 Chronic obstructive pulmonary disease		4	9	6			
DX7 History of prostate cancer		V	1	0		4	6

CPT CODES

PP1 Aphakic penetrating keratoplasty	6	5	7	5	0–LT
PR2 Posterior chamber intraocular lens scleral implant	6	6	9	8	5–LT
PR3 Open-sky mechanical automated vitrectomy	6	7	0	1	0–LT
PR4					
PR5					
PR6					
PR7					

PATIENT 4*

ICD-9-CM CODES

PDX Torn lateral meniscus of the right knee		8	3	6	.	1	
DX2 Torn anterior cruciate ligament of the right knee		8	4	4	.	2	
DX3					.		
DX4					.		

CPT CODES

PP1 Resection of tear of the lateral meniscus posterior horn	2	9	8	8	1–RT
PR2 Reconstruction of the anterior cruciate ligament using patellar tendon graft	2	9	8	8	8–RT
PR3					
PR4					
PR5					
PR6					
PR7					

*Please note that the answer sheets for CCS exam outpatient records require only 4 diagnoses and 7 procedures.

PATIENT 5

PDX Bunion (Please note the hypertrophy is not coded because this is inherent in a bunion.)

DX2

DX3

DX4

ICD-9-CM CODES

	7	2	7	.	1	
				.		
				.		
				.		

PP1
Bunionectomy with osteotomy

PR2

PR3

PR4

PR5

PR6

PR7

CPT CODES

2	8	2	9	6–TA

PATIENT 6*

ICD-9-CM CODES

PDX Laceration left ear lobe		8	7	2	.	0	1
DX2					.		
DX3					.		
DX4					.		

CPT CODES

PP1 Simple repair 2 cm laceration of ear lobe (2 cm laceration specified in the physical examination)	1	2	0	1	1–LT
PR2 E/M code based on Mapping Scenario provided (40 total points*)	9	9	2	8	3–25
PR3					
PR4					
PR5					
PR6					
PR7					

*According to the mapping scenario; meds given are = 1= 5 points, the history is problem focused = 10 points, the exam is problem focused = 10 points, the number of tests = 0 = 5 points, supplies = 2 suture kits = 10 points. This equals a total of 40 points.

PATIENT 7*

ICD-9-CM CODES

PDX Fracture humeral shaft		8	1	2	.	2	1
DX2 Smoking		3	0	5	.	1	
DX3					.		
DX4					.		

CPT CODES

PP1 Reduction of humeral shaft fracture (in CPT this would be called treatment of fracture with manipulation and casting)	2	4	5	0	5–LT
PR2 E/M code based on Mapping Scenario provided (50 total points)	9	9	2	8	4–25
PR3					
PR4					
PR5					
PR6					
PR7					

*According to the mapping scenario; meds given are = 2 = 5 points, the history is problem focused = 10 points, the exam is extended problem focused = 15 points, the number of tests = 5 = 15 points, supplies = 1 fracture tray = 5 points. This equals a total of 50 points.

PATIENT 8*

ICD-9-CM CODES

PDX Asthma with exacerbation		4	9	3	.	9	2
DX2					.		
DX3					.		
DX4					.		

CPT CODES

PP1 E/M code based on Mapping Scenario provided (36 total points)	9	9	2	8	4–25
PR2 Intravenous infusion	9	0	7	6	5
PR3					
PR4					
PR5					
PR6					
PR7					

*According to the mapping scenario; meds given are = 2 = 5 points, the history is problem focused = 10 points, the exam is extended problem focused = 15 points, the number of tests = 4 = 15 points, supplies = one venipuncture set and one intravenous set = 10 points. This equals a total of 55 points.

Patients 9 A and B

PATIENT 9 A

ICD-9-CM CODES

PDX Arteriosclerotic heart disease		4	1	4	.	0	1
DX2					.		
DX3					.		
DX4					.		

CPT CODES

PP1 Rt and Lt heart catheterization	9	3	5	2	6
PR2 Injection procedure for left angiography	9	3	5	4	3
PR3 Injection for aortography	9	3	5	4	4
PR4 Imaging supervision of cardiac catheterization and angiography	9	3	5	5	5
PR5 Imaging supervision of aortography	9	3	5	5	6
PR6 Coronary angiography	9	3	5	4	5
PR7					

PATIENT 9 B

ICD-9-CM CODES

PDX Arteriosclerotic heart disease		4	1	4	.	0	1
DX2					.		
DX3					.		
DX4					.		

CPT CODES

PP1 Transcatheter placement of an intracoronary stent(s), percutaneous, with or without other therapeutic intervention, any method; single vessel	9	2	9	8	0–LD
PR2 Left heart catheterizations	9	3	5	1	0
PR3 Coronary angiography	9	3	5	4	5
PR4 Left ventriculography	9	3	5	4	3
PR5					
PR6					
PR7					

Patients 10 A and B

PATIENT 10 A

ICD-9-CM CODES

PDX Metastatic carcinoma of liver		1	9	7	.	7	
DX2 Carcinoma of the lung		1	6	2	.	9	
DX3					.		
DX4					.		

CPT CODES

PP1 Percutaneous liver fine-needle biopsy	4	7	0	0	0
PR2 Ultrasound guidance	7	6	9	4	2
PR3					
PR4					
PR5					
PR6					
PR7					

PATIENT 10 B

ICD-9-CM CODES

PDX Chronic pain syndrome		3	3	8	.	4	
DX2 Lumbar radiculopathy		7	2	4	.	4	
DX3					.		
DX4					.		

CPT CODES

PP1 Injection, single (not via indwelling catheter), not including neurolytic substances, with or without contrast (for either localization or epidurography), of diagnostic or therapeutic substance(s) (including anesthetic, antispasmodic, opioid, steroid, other solution), epidural or subarachnoid; lumbar, sacral (caudal)	6	2	3	1	1
PR2 Injection single lumbar/sacral (see description above)	6	2	3	1	1–59
PR3 Injection single lumbar/sacral (see description above)	6	2	3	1	1–59
PR4					
PR5					
PR6					
PR7					

Patients 11 A and B

PATIENT 11 A

ICD-9-CM CODES

PDX Pain management		3	3	8	.	3	
DX2 Breast cancer of left upper lobe		1	7	4	.	8	
DX3 Metastatic bone CA		1	9	8	.	5	
DX4					.		

CPT CODES

PP1 Implantation programmable pump for pain management	6	2	3	6	2
PR2					
PR3					
PR4					
PR5					
PR6					
PR7					

PATIENT 11 B

ICD-9-CM CODES

PDX Reflex sympathetic dystrophy, left knee		3	3	7	.	2	2
DX2					.		
DX3					.		
DX4					.		

CPT CODES

PP1 Left lumbar sympathetic block with C-arm	6	4	5	2	0–LT
PR2 Fluroscopic guidance and localization of needle or catheter tip	7	7	0	0	3
PR3					
PR4					
PR5					
PR6					
PR7					

Answers for Part II: Inpatient Cases (Patients 12–21)

Answer sheets for CCS Examination inpatient records require only 10 diagnoses and 6 procedures.

PATIENT 12*

ICD-9-CM CODES

PDX Intertrochanteric fracture of femur		8	2	0	.	2	1
DX2 Postoperative urinary retention		9	9	7	.	5	
DX3 Urinary retention		7	8	8	.	2	0
DX4 Congestive heart failure		4	2	8	.	0	
DX5 Diverticulosis		5	6	2	.	1	0
DX6 Mitral regurgitation		4	2	4	.	0	
DX7 Coronary artery disease with ASHD		4	1	4	.	0	1
DX8 History of gastric ulcer disease		V	1	2	.	7	1
DX9 Degenerative joint disease		7	1	5	.	9	0
DX10 Dementia		2	9	0	.	1	0

ICD-9-CM CODES

PP1 Open reduction with internal fixation of femur	7	9	.	3	5
PR2			.		
PR3			.		
PR4			.		
PR5			.		
PR6			.		

*Note the CCS scoring sheet only provides space for 10 diagnoses and 6 procedures.

Notes on Patient 12

820.21 Radiology report denotes intertrochanteric fracture

997.5

788.20 Patient had postoperative urinary retention as documented in the Progress Note of 12/1. The 997 category directs us to use an additional code to identify the specific complication in addition to the 997 code. (See *Coding Clinic,* 2nd Quarter, 1998.)

428.0

562.10

424.0

414.01

V12.71

715.90

290.10

Please see Coding Practice section of this book: "Do not code 57.94 (Foley catheter)".

Points of Interest on Patient 12

1. One of the commonly missed complications is postoperative urinary retention. This case provides an example of this clinical scenario.
2. You must review the radiology report to determine where the fracture is. This is frequently the case with coding actual records.

PATIENT 12 A

ICD-9-CM CODES

PDX Delivery complicated by nuchal cord without compression		6	6	3	.	3	1
DX2 Outcome of newborn		V	2	7	.	0	
DX3 Mitral valve prolapse in pregnancy		6	4	8	.	6	1
DX4 Mitral valve prolapse		4	2	4	.	0	
DX5					.		
DX6					.		
DX7					.		
DX8					.		
DX9					.		
DX10					.		

ICD-9-CM CODES

PP1 Episiotomy with repair	7	3	.	6	
PR2			.		
PR3			.		
PR4			.		
PR5			.		
PR6			.		

Notes on Patient 12 A

663.31 This is a delivery with a nuchal cord wrapped around the baby's neck as per the delivery note.

V27.0 Outcome of delivery code

648.61 and 424.0 must be coded because it affected the monitoring of the patient and was documented in the medical record.

73.6 Episiotomy with repair

Points of Interest on Patient 12 A

1. This case is typical of many delivery charts in terms of documentation. Many times the practitioners document the complication of delivery in only one area such as the Delivery Note or the Operative Report. In this case, the baby has a nuchal cord but it is only mentioned once in the Delivery Record.
2. This is also an illustration of the three types of codes, at a minimum, that must be on every delivery chart: a diagnostic code from the delivery or pregnancy category, an outcome of birth code (V code), and a procedure code.

PATIENT 13

ICD-9-CM CODES

PDX Gram-negative pneumonia	4	8	2	.	8	3
DX2 Noninsulin-dependent diabetes (insulin requiring) out of control	2	5	0	.	5	2
DX3 Retinopathy	3	6	2	.	0	1
DX4 Hypertension	4	0	1	.	9	
DX5 Resistant gram-negative bacteria	V	0	9	.	2	
DX6 Degenerative joint disease of knees	7	1	5	.	3	6
DX7 Aortic stenosis	4	2	4	.	1	
DX8 Long-term use of insulin	V	5	8	.	6	7
DX9				.		
DX10				.		

ICD-9-CM CODES

PP1			.		
PR2			.		
PR3			.		
PR4			.		
PR5			.		
PR6			.		

Notes on Patient 13

482.83 Gram-negative pneumonia documented on H & P and Progress Note of 2/2. (*Coding Clinic* 3rd Quarter 1988.)

250.52 Noninsulin-dependent diabetes mellitus (insulin requiring) used because the H & P states "Diabetes Mellitus—uncontrolled" 1/31 Progress Note addresses treatment plan for poor control. Orders of 1/31 and 2/1 reflect treatment. The blood glucose record reflects high blood sugar. (See *Coding Clinic* 4th Quarter, 1997, 2nd Quarter 1997, 2nd Quarter 2002, 3rd Quarter 2002.)

V58.67 Long-term use of insulin

362.01 Retinopathy documented on the Discharge Summary

401.9 Documented on the H & P and Discharge Summary. The patient is on HCTZ for this condition

V09.2 Used because the resistant organism is documented in the Discharge Summary and the laboratory reports. Furthermore, the patient was tried on erythromycin and needed to be changed to another antibiotic.

715.36 Documented in the D/C Summary, H & P and the orders

424.1 Documented in the D/C Summary, H & P and in the orders

Points of Interest on Patient 13

1. The patient has pneumonia and we need to have the organism causing the pneumonia specified in the medical record in areas other than just the sputum culture.
2. The patient also has uncontrolled diabetes as evidenced by the labile blood sugar and the documentation in the record.
3. According to basic ICD coding books, you should only use the V codes denoting resistance when the resistance is documented by the physician(s) involved.

PATIENT 13 A

ICD-9-CM CODES

PDX Intrauterine death		6	5	6	.	4	1
DX2 Cephalopelvic disproportion		6	5	3	.	4	1
DX3 Nuchal cord without compression		6	6	3	.	3	1
DX4 Delivery with obesity		6	4	9	.	1	1
DX5 Obesity		2	7	8	.	0	0
DX6 Stillborn		V	2	7	.	1	
DX7					.		
DX8					.		
DX9					.		
DX10					.		

ICD-9-CM CODES

PP1 C-section	7	4	.	0	
PR2 Artificial rupture of membranes (not for induction of labor)	7	3	.	0	9
PR3 Fetal monitor	7	5	.	3	2
PR4			.		
PR5			.		
PR6			.		

Notes on Patient 13 A

656.41 Intrauterine death of the baby

653.41 Cephalopelvic disproportion

663.31 Used to denote the nuchal cord without compression as documented in the operative report

649.11 Obesity in pregnancy and delivery

278.00

V27.1 Outcome of delivery for stillborn code

74.0 Cesarean section

73.09 Used to denote the artificial rupture of membranes performed after Pitocin is administered and labor fails to progress as documented in the H & P.

75.32 Use of internal fetal monitor.

See the Coding Practice section of this book: "Code all procedures that fall within the code range 01.01–86.99, but do not code 57.94 (Foley catheter)."

Points of Interest on Patient 13 A

This is an example of a very unfortunate situation of a baby's death. The intrauterine death is sequenced first because it is the reason for the Cesarean section. Although it was thought that the patient had cephalopelvic disproportion, the urgency of undertaking the Cesarean section was due to the lack of fetal heart tones.

PATIENT 14

ICD-9-CM CODES

PDX Admission for chemotherapy		V	5	8	.	1	1
DX2 Carcinomatosis with malignant ascites		1	9	7	.	6	
DX3 History of colon carcinoma (organ removed)		V	1	0	.	0	5
DX4 Status colostomy		V	4	4	.	3	
DX5 Family history of colon cancer		V	1	6	.	0	
DX6 History of radiation therapy		V	1	5	.	3	
DX7 Malignant ascites		7	8	9	.	5	1
DX8 History of tobacco abuse		V	1	5	.	8	2
DX9					.		
DX10					.		

ICD-9-CM CODES

PP1 Chemotherapy	9	9	.	2	5
PR2			.		
PR3			.		
PR4			.		
PR5			.		
PR6			.		

Notes on Patient 14

V58.11 The patient is admitted for chemotherapy. This is documented in the Discharge Summary and is reflected in the Physician Orders.

197.6 Carcinomatosis with malignant ascites documented on the Discharge Summary and in the H & P.

789.51 Malignant ascites.

Note: The ICD-9-CM tabular index requires that the malignancy be coded first.

V10.05 The organ of origin (colon) has been removed; therefore, code the history of malignant neoplasm of the colon. Whenever there is a secondary neoplasm code, you need to have a primary site designated either with a code for the primary site or a V code. If the primary site for the neoplasm is not known, use code 199.1.

V44.3 Status colostomy is reflected on the H & P.

V16.0 Relevant to the patient's treatment and is documented in the medical record.

Note: The breast cyst is not coded because it does not meet UHDDS criteria.

99.25 See the Coding Practice section of this book: the code for chemotherapy (99.25) would be assigned.

Points of Interest on Patient 14

1. This case illustrates several basic principles of coding neoplasms. First, the patient had the organ in which the carcinoma arose removed (organ of origin). Second, because you are coding a secondary site, you must code the primary in some manner. Therefore, use a history of malignant code (V10.06) to represent the primary site.
2. This case also illustrates that when the ascites is determined to have malignant cells in the fluid, you use the code for malignant ascites.

PATIENT 15

ICD-9-CM CODES

PDX	Recurrent lung carcinoma		1	6	2	.	5	
DX2	Intraoperative MI		9	9	7	.	1	
DX3	Nontransmural MI		4	1	0	.	7	1
DX4	Hypertension		4	0	1	.	9	
DX5	Iatrogenic hypotension		4	5	8	.	2	9
DX6	COPD		4	9	6	.		
DX7	DJD of lumbar spine		7	2	1	.	3	
DX8	Hemiparesis of dominant side late effect of stroke		4	3	8	.	2	1
DX9	History of tobacco abuse		V	1	5	.	8	2
DX10	Surgical absence lung		V	4	5	.	7	6

ICD-9-CM CODES

PP1	Pneumonectomy	3	2	.	5	9
PR2				.		
PR3				.		
PR4				.		
PR5				.		
PR6				.		

Notes on Patient 15

162.5	Recurrent lung cancer is documented in the H & P, Discharge Summary, and the operative report
997.1	Intraoperative myocardial infarction (MI)
410.71	Postoperative/intraoperative myocardial infarction is documented in the Progress Notes
401.9	Hypertension documented in the H & P and in the D/C Summary
458.29	Would be coded because this is the precipitating factor causing the MI

496, 721.3, 438.21, V15.82, V45.76: Would be coded because they are documented in the medical record and are relevant to the admission

32.59	The pneumonectomy is documented in the operative report

Points of Interest on Patient 15

In this case you practice coding an intraoperative complication. Further, you need to differentiate if the myocardial infarction caused the hypotension or if the hypotension caused the myocardial infarction. In this case, the intraoperative hypotension occurred, which resulted in an MI. This case illustrates that problem. This is a clinical scenario about which coders have had little education.

PATIENT 16*

ICD-9-CM CODES

PDX Acute inferior MI initial episode		4	1	0	.	4	1
DX2 Complete heart block		4	2	6	.	0	
DX3 Hematemesis		5	7	8	.	0	
DX4 Acute blood loss anemia		2	8	5	.	1	
DX5 Hyperlipidemia		2	7	2	.	4	
DX6 Arteriosclerotic coronary artery disease		4	1	4	.	0	1
DX7 Nausea and vomiting		7	8	7	.	0	1
DX8 Adverse effect of anesthetics	E	9	3	8	.	4	
DX9 History of tobacco use		V	1	5	.	8	2
DX10					.		

ICD-9-CM CODES

PP1 CABG × 2	3	6	.	1	2
PR2 Insertion of nondrug-eluting stent(s)	3	6	.	0	6
PR3 Left heart catheterization	3	7	.	2	2
PR4 Angiography	8	8	.	5	5
PR5 Ventriculography	8	8	.	5	3
PR6 EGD	4	5	.	1	3

The following procedures would *not* be coded: "Code all procedures that fall within the code range through 86.99, but do not code 57.94 (Foley catheter)." (Refer to the Coding Practice section of this book.)

PTCA	0	0		6	6
Insertion of one vascular stent	0	0		4	5
Procedure on single vessel	0	0		4	0

*Note that only 6 procedures are to be coded but Extracorporeal circulation and TPA should be coded if there were room as well.

Notes on Patient 16

410.41 Acute inferior MI is documented on the 4/20 EKG. This is also evident from the laboratory reports. The CK-MB is elevated.

426.0 Complete heart block is documented on the discharge summary and the H & P as well as the EKG.

530.7

578.0

787.01

E938.4

You would code the hematemesis because no cause has been found. The nausea and vomiting is the adverse effect of a drug.

285.1 Following the upper gastrointestinal bleeding, the patient experienced acute blood loss anemia.

414.01 The patient is found to have arteriosclerotic heart disease. Code the native artery (fifth digit of one) because the patient has never undergone bypass surgery prior to this admission. Therefore, assume that the ASHD is of the native artery.

272.4 Hyperlipidemia is documented on the H & P and the Summary.

V15.82 History of tobacco use

36.12 CABG 3 2

36.01 PTCA

36.06 Insertion stent

37.22 Left heart cath

88.55 Angiography using a single catheter

88.53 Ventriculography

45.13 EGD

39.61 Extracorporeal circulation

Points of Interest on Patient 16

1. You must code the site of the myocardial infarction to obtain the correct fourth digit. In order to do this, look at the EKG to determine the site of acute inferior myocardial infarction.
2. This case also requires that you code the upper gastrointestinal hemorrhage because there is no specified cause.
3. Recognize that the nausea and vomiting is an adverse effect of anesthesia.
4. The CABG and the heart catheterization provide practice in this area. Remember stents, if they are placed, with an additional code when coding PTCAs. You also need to code the angiography and ventriculography, if done. To correctly code these procedures, the coder must carefully determine how many catheters are used during angiography in order to code them appropriately.
5. If extracorporeal circulation is used, you should code this as directed by the ICD-9-CM codebook notation. You would not code cardioplegia because this is included in the coronary artery bypass code.

PATIENT 17

ICD-9-CM CODES

PDX *E coli* septicemia		0	3	8	.	4	2
DX2 Acute pyelonephritis		5	9	0	.	1	0
DX3 Herpes simplex		0	5	4	.	9	
DX4 Resistant organism to Penicillin and Ampicillin		V	0	9	.	0	
DX5 Tobacco abuse		3	0	5	.	1	
DX6 Family history of diabetes		V	1	8	.	0	
DX7					.		
DX8					.		
DX9					.		
DX10					.		

ICD-9-CM CODES

PP1			.		
PR2			.		
PR3			.		
PR4			.		
PR5			.		
PR6			.		

Notes on Patient 17

038.42 *E coli* septicemia is documented on the culture and sensitivity as well as in the Discharge Summary. Note: SIRS is not used here because septicemia is documented (versus sepsis).

590.10 Acute pyelonephritis is also coded because this is where the septicemia began. Do not code the organism as per guidelines in the *Coding Clinic* 4th Quarter 1988. It is already reflected in the septicemia code.

054.9 Herpes simplex is documented on the 9/8 progress notes and is treated.

305.1 Tobacco abuse is treated and documented in the progress notes, H & P and D/C summary. Note that 305.1 does not require a 5th digit (ICD-9-CM codebook tabular index).

The pyelogram performed on 9/8 is *not* coded because it is an unspecified pyelogram. See the Coding Practice section of this book a pyelogram is coded only if it is code 87.74 or 87.76 (Retrogrades, urinary systems).

V09.0 The organism is specified to be resistant to in the discharge summary and therefore designate that in the coding.

Points of Interest on Patient 17

1. This case illustrates how an infection can begin in one organ system and then become systemic. This is why you find the same organism in the urinary tract as in the blood. As stated earlier, code both disorders (septicemia and pyelonephritis).
2. The organism causing the infection is resistant to penicillin and ampicillin. You only code resistance to a drug if the resistance is documented by the practitioner in the record. Do not code from the laboratory reports alone.

PATIENT 18

ICD-9-CM CODES

PDX	Dehydration		2	7	6	.	5	1
DX2	Diarrhea due to Sinemet		7	8	7	.	9	1
DX3	Adverse reaction to Sinemet	E	9	3	6	.	4	
DX4	Parkinson's disease		3	3	2	.	0	
DX5	Esophageal reflux		5	3	0	.	8	1
DX6	Hypertension with chronic kidney disease		4	0	3	.	9	1
DX7	CHF		4	2	8	.	0	
DX8	Chronic kidney disease		5	8	5	.	9	
DX9						.		
DX10						.		

ICD-9-CM CODES

PP1			.		
PR2			.		
PR3			.		
PR4			.		
PR5			.		
PR6			.		

Notes on Patient 18

276.51 Dehydration is documented in the H & P and the Discharge Summary.

787.91 Diarrhea due to Sinemet *(Coding Clinic* 3rd Quarter 1995, 10)

Note: The diarrhea and dehydration are both treated. Sequence 276.51 first because this code optimizes the case in the setting of MS-DRGs.

E936.4 Adverse reaction to Sinemet

The following are documented in the Discharge Summary:

332.0 Parkinson's disease

530.81 Esophageal reflux

428.0 This condition is documented in the medical record and is treated.

403.91 and 585.9 Note that Coding Guidelines require that both the combination hypertension code and chronic kidney disease

Points of Interest on Patient 18

1. The crux of coding this case revolves around the adverse reaction to Sinemet. This is somewhat challenging in that Sinemet is not in the ICD-9-CM codebook. It is, however, a very common anti-Parkinson's drug. An experienced coder should know this drug is associated with this disease and subsequently understand how to code an adverse effect.
2. This case also illustrates an optimization issue. Both the dehydration and diarrhea (the adverse effect) are treated. Therefore, two diagnoses equally meet the definition of principal diagnosis. Sequence the one that provides the highest DRG first as the principal diagnosis.

PATIENT 19

ICD-9-CM CODES

PDX ITP		2	8	7	.	3	1
DX2 Cirrhosis of the liver		5	7	1	.	2	
DX3 Type I diabetes mellitus		2	5	0	.	0	1
DX4 Chronic alcoholism		3	0	3	.	9	3
DX5 ASHD		4	1	4	.	0	0
DX6 Post-op respiratory distress		5	1	8	.	5	
DX7 Hyperlipidemia		2	7	2	.	4	
DX8 Hypertension		4	0	1	.	9	
DX9 s/p CABG		V	4	5	.	8	1
DX10 History of TIA		V	1	2	.	8	2

ICD-9-CM CODES

PP1 Splenectomy	4	1	.	5	
PR2 Ventilator management	9	6	.	7	1
PR3 Insertion endotracheal tube	9	6	.	0	4
PR4 Point of interest: 99.05 transfusion platelet and 99.04 transfusion of PRBC on reference page			.		
PR5			.		
PR6			.		

Notes on Patient 19

287.31 Idiopathic thrombocytopenic purpura—documented in the H & P and the Discharge Summary.

571.2

250.01

303.93

414.00

518.5 Postoperative respiratory distress is documented in the 6/24 Progress Notes.

272.4

401.9

V45.81

These conditions are documented on the Discharge Summary and/or the H & P.

41.5 Splenectomy documented on the operative report

96.71 Ventilator management begun on 6/24

96.04 Insertion endotracheal tube

Points of Interest on Patient 19

1. As is evident from the documentation, this case provides practice coding respiratory distress following surgery.
2. This case also provides the opportunity to code alcoholism and a related physical condition.

PATIENT 20

ICD-9-CM CODES

PDX Congestive heart failure		4	2	8	.	0	
DX2 Tricuspid insufficiency		3	9	7	.	0	
DX3 Type I diabetes		2	5	0	.	0	1
DX4 Mycotic nails		1	1	0	.	1	
DX5 Hypertrophic nails		7	0	3	.	8	
DX6 Hypertension		4	0	1	.	9	
DX7 Tobacco abuse		3	0	5	.	1	
DX8					.		
DX9					.		
DX10					.		

ICD-9-CM CODES

PP1 Débridement of mycotic nails × 2	8	6	.	2	7
PR2	8	6	.	2	7
PR3			.		
PR4			.		
PR5			.		
PR6			.		

Notes on Patient 20

428.0 The patient is admitted with CHF. This is documented on the H & P and Discharge Summary. Even though the patient also has mitral and aortic valve insufficiency, use the 428.0 because, as per *Coding Clinic* 2nd Quarter 2000, there is no documentation that the CHF is rheumatic.

397.0 Tricuspid insufficiency is documented on the Discharge Summary and H & P.

250.01 Diabetes mellitus type I is documented on the Discharge Summary and H & P.

110.1 Mycotic nails, 703.8 Hypertrophic nails, 401.9 Hypertension, 305.1 Tobacco abuse are all documented in the medical record and meet the UHDDS definition. Note that 305.1 does not require a 5th digit (ICD-9-CM codebook tabular index).

The podiatric consultation documented these conditions.

86.27 Débridement of nails performed as per the progress notes and the consult sheet. Refer to the Coding Practice section of this book, "Code all procedures that fall within the code range 01.01–86.99, but do not code 57.94 (Foley catheter)." This is coded twice because it is a bilateral débridement.

Points of Interest on Patient 20

1. This case provides an example of the coding rules for coding congestive heart failure with a heart valve disorder (*Coding Clinic* 2nd Quarter 2000).
2. The documentation provided also is interesting. The only place that the procedure is documented is in the consultation. This is a practice in some healthcare facilities and illustrates the need to review every document in the record in order to code accurately.

PATIENT 21

ICD-9-CM CODES

PDX Incomplete abortion with hemorrhage		6	3	4	.	1	1
DX2 Pregnancy complicated by abuse		6	4	9	.	0	3
DX3 Pregnancy complicated by alcohol abuse		6	4	8	.	4	3
DX4 Depression		3	1	1	.		
DX5 Alcohol abuse		3	0	5	.	0	1
DX6					.		
DX7					.		
DX8					.		
DX9					.		
DX10					.		

ICD-9-CM CODES

PP1 Dilatation and curettage following spontaneous abortion	6	9	.	0	2
PR2			.		
PR3			.		
PR4			.		
PR5			.		
PR6			.		

Notes on Patient 21

634.11 This is a case of an incomplete spontaneous abortion. This is evidenced by the Pathology Report. (See *Coding Clinic* 4th Quarter 1995.) The patient has documented heavy bleeding that has resulted in anemia. Therefore, use the fourth digit of 1 and a fifth digit of 1.

648.43, 305.01 Alcohol abuse is treated and relevant to the case. The physician documented that the patient had "alcohol abuse", even though clinically the patient may have alcoholism. Therefore, alcohol abuse, the diagnosis that is documented, is the one that is coded (*Coding Clinic* 2nd Quarter, 1998). As per coding guidelines the 648.43 is used as well as codes 311 and 305.01 that add further specificity.

649.03 Tobacco abuse is also documented and treated. The pregnancy (649.03) code is specific to tobacco abuse and because of this we only use the one code.

69.02 The patient underwent a D & C following spontaneous abortion.

Points of Interest on Patient 21

This case illustrated the difference between coding an incomplete spontaneous abortion and a complication of abortion. In the documentation of the record you are told the patient has had a D & C to complete the spontaneous abortion. You may therefore think that this should be coded with a code from the 639 category. However, if there are products of conception or other material from the pregnancy retained in the uterus at the time of readmission, this indicates that the abortion was not completed. Therefore, use the 634 category. If, on the other hand, there was no retained material, use the 639 category (complication of spontaneous abortion). Please note that spontaneous abortion and miscarriage are used interchangeably in ICD-9-CM.